HEREDITY AND YOU

Also by the Author

TEEN-AGE MEDICINE: *Questions Young People
Ask About Their Health*

HEREDITY
AND
YOU

How You Can Protect
Your Family's Future

by

Augusta Greenblatt
with Foreword by Leon E. Rosenberg, MD

COWARD, McCANN & GEOGHEGAN, INC.
NEW YORK

SBN: 698-10588-5

Library of Congress Catalog Card Number: 73-93773

PRINTED IN THE UNITED STATES OF AMERICA

For my mother and father, Rissi and Raful Pecker, who taught me that man inherits more than his genes from his parents

Contents

Acknowledgments

The story of heredity and health is more than a collection of medical observations and scientific facts. It is the story of the families to whom genetic diseases happen, the doctors who are helping them cope with the realities of today, and the scientists who are giving them new hopes for tomorrow.

Without their generosity in sharing their agonies and their triumphs the book could not have been written.

You may question why I included some diseases and omitted others. Admittedly the choices were not easy among the 2,000 genetic disorders identified to date. For the most part I tried to focus not only on disorders affecting relatively large numbers of individuals, but particularly on those for which concrete help is available now. The most difficult decision was the one to bypass coronary heart disease and some of its associated problems—hypertension, diabetes, gout, and obesity. The recurrent theme is: what can be prevented, what can be treated, what can be ameliorated.

While the scientists were most candid in acknowledging the magnitude of the problems still to be solved, they were at the same time infectious in their enthusiasm for the immense strides already made.

I am especially grateful to the following for their cooperation as a source of material as well as for their help in reviewing specific chapters. Any errors are mine alone.

Dr. Louis M. Aledort, Mount Sinai School of Medicine, Medical Director of the National Hemophilia Foundation; Dr. Richard Goodman, Department of Human Genetics, Medical School, The Sheba Medical Center, Tel-Hashomer, Israel; Joseph Mori, Science Information Division, National Foundation-March of Dimes; National Institute of Mental Health, Public Information Branch, Office of Communications; Dr. Howard Pearson, Professor of Pediatrics, Yale University School of Medicine; Dr. Leon E. Rosenberg, Chairman of the Department of Human Genetics, Yale University School of Medicine; Dr. Edward J. Schutta, Chief of the Section of Medical Genetics, Brookdale Hospital Medical Center, Brooklyn, New York; Dr. Edward C. Zaino, Medical Director of Cooley's Anemia Blood and Research Foundation. I also wish to thank Adele Berman, and Ida Kroll for their patience and secretarial skills.

Finally, my thanks to my editor, Peggy Brooks, for her unerring sensitivity to what is relevant and clear to you the reader.

Foreword

In his futuristic film *Sleeper*, Woody Allen proclaims his desire "to clone alone." This hilarious line fits perfectly in a zany story about life in the twenty-second century. Unfortunately, it too closely reflects the image that the field of human genetics has in the minds of today's public. In the past two years several writers have told me of their desire to write a book about human genetics for the layman, replete with such matters as test tube fertilization, mass cloning of good or evil men, and subjugation of civilizations through genetic manipulation. Although I believe deeply that the public must become better informed about the genetics of man, I discouraged each of these people because I feared that, in their hands, human genetics might be seen as an evil force for social control, and geneticists might be pictured as the high priests of this frightening scientific technocracy. That simply is not the way it is.

Human genetics is a very young field, born in this century,

11

infantile until only twenty years ago, and now undergoing a most impressive adolescent growth spurt. Much has been learned about the chemistry of the genetic material (DNA), the mechanisms by which it is copied from generation to generation, and the means by which it is packaged in microscopic bodies called chromosomes. Much, too, has been discovered about the processes which continually change man's genes. Such changes, called mutations, occur in minute number in each of us and account for the enormous diversity which typifies the human species. Most of these genetic alterations are harmless. Others are not, and as a medically trained human geneticist it is these deleterious mutations which confront me daily.

Almost 2,000 different human genetic disorders have been described, leading to major congenital aberrations in 3 percent of all live births and minor abnormalities in an additional 2 percent. In addition, as many as 4 percent of all pregnancies terminate in the first weeks after conception because of chromosomal anomalies in the embryo which are incompatible with prolonged life. Congenital and inherited disorders are the second leading cause of death in children and account for nearly a third of all pediatric admissions to hospitals.

It is this story of medical discovery and human suffering that Augusta Greenblatt has captured in her book *Heredity and You*. With painstaking care, she has described the biological basis of selected genetic disorders and their emotional impact on people. She has identified the moral and ethical arguments which society must confront surrounding such issues as genetic counseling, screening, and prenatal diagnosis. She has understood that medical genetics is aimed, not at the construction of some awesome brave new world, but at the prevention of disease and the detection and treatment of patients with inherited disorders. And, she has translated into clear prose the sometimes obscure and always technical language of the medical investigator. For these accom-

plishments Mrs. Greenblatt deserves the admiration and grati-
tude of the scientist and, more important, the readership of the
public at large.

LEON E. ROSENBERG, MD
Chairman, Department
of Human Genetics
Yale University School
of Medicine
New Haven, Connecticut

HEREDITY AND YOU

1

Unraveling the Mystery of Heredity

The time has not yet come when a "how to" book on genetics can promise you a child that will paint like Picasso, swim like Spitz, and think like Einstein. But if you are among the millions whose families are touched by hereditary disease, you can now be given new hope and reassurance.

As the mystery of heredity is unraveled, answers begin to emerge: for the parents of an affected child who ask, "Why did it happen to us and can it happen again?"; for the mother-to-be who wants to know during pregnancy if her unborn child is a victim; and for the healthy young people who fear for the future of their children because a hereditary disease is present in a relative.

Almost 2,000 genetic disorders have been identified to date, with new ones added to the medical literature at a steady rate. Some are very rare and affect only a handful of families. Others are clustered in particular ethnic groups including Tay-Sachs disease in Eastern European Jews, thalassemia in Greeks and Italians, and sickle cell disease in blacks.

Still other disorders, not categorized primarily as hereditary, are getting a closer look by doctors as the genetic components become more conspicuous. On the growing list are heart disease, high blood pressure, diabetes, obesity, mental illness, psoriasis, and even balding. Indeed when Emory University School of Medicine announced the First Human Hair Symposium in October, 1973, it included a presentation on "Genetics of Hair."

While it is not yet possible to cure genetic diseases, an increasing number of victims can now be successfully treated and ameliorated with medication and diet. Not the least of the good news is the realization that most genes, good and bad, simple and complex, depend to some degree on their environment for their expression. Are you born to be fat if both your parents are? Probably only if you start overeating with your first morsel in infancy and continue to stuff yourself as you grow. Are you born to be smart or stupid? A good deal may depend not only on your genes, but on your motivation, education, and experience. Defective and crippling genes need no longer be the ruling destiny to all who bear them.

From the time man first recognized his capacity to pass on his characteristics to his offspring, he has wrestled with the puzzle of heredity and reproduction. When Hippocrates in the fourth century B.C. observed that "bald people are descended from bald people, people with blue eyes from people with blue eyes, and squinting persons from squinting persons," he cautiously added, "at least in the majority of cases." He was at a loss to explain such obvious exceptions as the blue-eyed children of brown-eyed parents.

A few hundred years later Talmudic scholars were closer to the mark with their description of a genetic disease that caused male infants in certain families to bleed dangerously at circumcision. They had a fine description of hemophilia, but it was an isolated phenomenon.

As recently as the beginning of the eighteenth century some scientists thought there was a fully formed little man or woman in each female egg. The only function of the sperm, they maintained, was to trigger the egg to start the little man growing. Other scientists, offended by the small role assigned to the male, contended that the little man (homunculus) is actually in the sperm and injected into the egg at conception.

Fanciful as this may sound, the correct explanation is even more bizarre—that your life begins with a single cell to which your mother and father have each contributed the information that will make you uniquely you and at the same time unmistakably their offspring. Within that single cell is enough information to fill forty-six encyclopedic volumes of more than 15,000 pages each. The language of heredity uses only four letters (call them AGCT for the present), three-letter words, and a code that can be read and translated by all forms of life—bacteria, fruit flies, sweet peas, fleas, mice, and men. Scientists believe that the same code has been in continuous use for more than 3.5 billion years.

The substance in which the information is stored is DNA (deoxyribonucleic acid), an immensely thin, long molecule with extraordinary properties. If all your DNA were uncoiled, it could span a distance equal to the diameter of the solar system. Yet DNA occupies so little space that the genetic information for all people alive on earth today could easily fit into a large drop of water.

We also know how the information is transmitted from one generation to the next with almost flawless accuracy, what happens when a mistake is made and the message comes through garbled, and how the information is used to direct the complex and orderly processes of life itself.

Most of the knowledge about genetics has been acquired with an explosive momentum in the last twenty years. The revelations have inspired both admiration and fear. Do we now have the power to create life from chemicals on the laboratory shelf? (As recently as the fall of 1973 a Massachusetts Institute of Technology Nobel Laureate announced the successful synthesis of an artificial gene that promises to behave biologically exactly like its natural counterpart.) How will we use the new power and who will make the decisions?

The fact is we have the power today not to create Frankenstein monsters, but to prevent them.

To understand how the new look of heredity came about and what it can mean in your future, it will help to become acquainted with the vocabulary of genetics. For the reader who is content at this point to know no more about DNA than that it would be a low-scoring Scrabble tile, you may safely skip some of the following passages and return when you choose. The reader who wants to go beyond the scope of this chapter will find a list of suggested readings on page 239.

The early days of modern genetics were marked by a number of brilliant discoveries, some of which were unfortunately received with either apathy or disbelief. Others were initially ignored only to be dusted off and appreciated decades later. Classical geneticists (botanists and zoologists) were often unaware of what was happening in the biochemist's laboratory, and both groups were unfamiliar with the early contributions of a few physicians concerned with human hereditary disease.

It all came together in recent years with a new breed of scientist—the molecular biologists. Using the tools and know-how of physics, mathematics, biology, biochemistry, and genetics, they found answers hitherto not possible. They also won an impressive number of Nobel prizes on the way.*

The first scientific clues to heredity came from a monastery garden in Austria a little more than a century ago. After repeat-

---

* George Beadle, Edward Tatum, Joshua Lederberg, Arthur Kornberg, Severo Ochoa, Francis Crick, James Watson, Maurice Wilkins, François Jacob, André Lwoff, Jacques Monod, Marshall Nirenberg, H. Gobind Khorana, Robert W. Holley, Max Delbrück, Alfred Hershey, Salvador E. Luria.

edly failing his exams to teach natural science in secondary school, Augustinian monk Gregor Mendel spent four semesters at the University of Vienna filling in the gaps in his science education. He plunged into his research fresh from his experiences with prominent astronomers, physicists, and mathematicians of the day.

Specifically Mendel set out to learn more about what happens when hybrid plants (offspring of parents with different characteristics) are bred. How do these characteristics show up in succeeding generations? Is there a pattern, and if so, can it be predicted? These are more or less the questions we ask about ourselves, for each of us is a hybrid—the product of two different individuals of the same species.

The homunculus (the preformed little man theory) was no longer on the scene in the middle 1850's. In his place was a belief that each part of the body contributes its qualities to the germ cells (the egg and sperm) and the offspring represents a blending of the characteristics of each parent at the time of conception.

The theory had some attractive features and even allowed acquired characteristics, such as a father's strong muscles or a mother's cooking skill, to be inherited. But it failed to explain why some children resembled their grandparents, aunts, and uncles more than their parents. As for bald fathers and sons, most fathers are not yet bald when their sons are conceived

For his experiments Mendel chose purebred specimens of sweet peas with a number of visible differences—red or white flowers, long or short stems, smooth or rough seeds. When he bred red with white, all the flowers in the first generation were red. Where had the white gone? He found that out when he bred the hybrids with each other. Their offspring were both red and white—in a proportion of three to one. The white was there all the time but seemed to skip a generation before it showed up again intact.

Mendel also noted that characteristics that appear together in one generation are transmitted independently in succeeding generations, so that long-stemmed red flowers bred with short-stemmed white flowers produced red and white flowers with either long or short stems.

After eight years of painstaking work with more than 8,000 plants Mendel published his well-documented results in 1865. In sharp contradiction to the prevailing view, he proposed that heredity is *not* a blending. Traits (he called them characters) are transmitted in separate independent units. Each character is controlled by a factor contributed by each parent (we call them genes and although that term did not come into use until the early part of the twentieth century, it will be convenient to take the liberty of using it now with apologies for taking it out of historical context).

Some traits such as red flowers, long stems, and smooth seeds are dominant and in each case can be transmitted by a single gene. Others, such as white flowers and short stems, are recessive and require a double dose of the gene.

The patterns Mendel set down from heredity in sweet peas apply to virtually every form of life, including man:

Each of your parents contributes equally to your inheritance.

For each physical character each parent contributes one gene.

The two genes may not be identical—one may say "brown eyes" the other "blue." Such alternative forms of the same gene are called alleles.

If you inherit two identical genes for one trait—two brown or two blue— you are homozygous for that trait.

If you inherit one of each, you are a heterozygote.

When the genes for a particular trait are not identical, one may dominate over the other—*i.e.*, only that one gene is needed for the trait to be expressed. Mendel's red flowers, long stems, and your brown eye gene are dominant. Other traits, such as those for white flowers and blue eyes, are recessive and need a double dose of the gene to show up.

Your genotype is the sum of your genes. Your phenotype is the various characteristic expressed by your genotype.

When you inherit a gene for brown eyes from each of your parents, you are homozygous and your eyes are brown. You may, however, inherit brown from one parent and blue from the other. You are a heterozygote, but your eyes will still be brown. The gene for blue is still there. Your brown-eyed mate may also be a heterozygote for eye color. In every pregnancy each of you, purely by chance, may transmit the gene for blue (the probability is one in four). The baby with a double dose for blue eyes is the blue-eyed offspring of brown-eyed parents that puzzled the ancients.

While the rules are the same for Mendel's sweet peas and man, the game is different. The traits he studied are controlled by a single gene. Few of ours are. Many of our most interesting characteristics are polygenic (controlled by a number of genes) —stature, skin color, intelligence, mental illness. Moreover, Mendel had a tight control over the conditions in which his plants grew. In man, even identical twins, especially those reared apart, differ in weight, height, IQ, and many other traits in which environment counts.

Application of Mendel's laws to man made it possible to explain for the first time how perfectly healthy parents can produce one or more children with severe genetic defects. Tay-Sachs disease, PKU, galactosemia, sickle cell disease, and others described in other sections of the book require a double dose of a defective gene to inflict their damage. If you have one good gene for the trait and one defective gene, you are a carrier, but your good gene will protect you. If your mate is also a carrier and each of you transmits your defective gene, your child, with a double dose, has no such protection.

Whether the good or the bad gene is transmitted is purely a matter of chance, but it is no longer a matter of chance today to identify a carrier in advance. Carriers of a defective recessive gene can transmit it for many generations, and there will be no hint of its presence until a child is born to two carriers. Such grim surprises can now be avoided for many. In dozens of disorders individuals who are afraid they are at risk either because the disease has already appeared somewhere in the family or because they are members of an ethnic group with a high concentration of carriers can be tested and warned in advance.

When a disease is caused by a dominant gene (only one dose of the gene required), each offspring has a fifty-fifty chance of inheriting it from his affected parent. Even the other parent's normal gene is no protection. The child who inherits the affected parent's normal gene is of course safe from the disease. The chain of inheritance is broken. He is not a carrier, and his children are safe.

A few years after Mendel's publication a twenty-two-year-old family physician in Long Island was to describe the precise pattern of inheritance of a dominant gene in one of the most devastating of all hereditary disorders—Huntington's chorea (Chapter 16).

When young Dr. George Huntington nailed down the genetic basis of the disease, he knew nothing of Mendel's work. Nor was that surprising. What was surprising was that Mendel's fellow geneticists and botanists knew just as little. Contrary to the waves Mendel's discoveries should have made, they barely created a ripple. Although the journal in which his paper was published was sent to 120 libraries, virtually no one was impressed. Mendel seemed consigned to oblivion.

There is a special irony in Mendel's failure to gain recognition at the time. It was the period when the intellectual, scientific, and religious world was rocked by Charles Darwin's *Origin of Species,* suggesting that the earth and all life on it had not appeared ready-made but that various species evolved from common ancestors by imperceptible changes over millions of generations. Darwin needed a good theory of heredity, but he died sixteen years after Mendel's work was completed without ever having heard of the botanist monk.

"My time will come," Mendel commented bitterly. It came thirty-five years later when he was rediscovered in 1900. Today his name is in every dictionary, biology, and genetics book, and his contributions are universally recognized as the earliest and still valid milestones in the science of heredity.

Mendel's concern was with the how of heredity rather than with the material responsible for it. If genes are transmitted as separate units in an orderly manner, there should be identifiable bits of matter serving as vehicles for the genes. By the last half of the nineteenth century it was already known that the cell is the basic unit of life and all living cells come from other living cells. Each cell, we now know, is a very intricate and busy chemical factory. It has raw materials from which it builds its own complex molecules, it has a source of energy, and it thrives and grows until it is ready to divide. The body is constantly replacing many of its cells—skin, liver, blood, etc. When the division takes place, each daughter cell is identical with the mother cell from which it originates.

Within the cell is a dense demarcated region, the nucleus, Here is where the control center is located. Remove the nucleus and the cell no longer lives, grows, or divides. With the development of organic dyes in the 1880's the nucleus began to reveal details of itself. What looks like a random jumble of threadlike bodies begin to undergo changes when the cell is ready to divide. The threads become shorter, plumper, and more discrete. Named chromosomes because they stain deeply with the dye, the threadlike bodies line up and each one makes an exact copy of itself before the cell divides. Each of the new cells now has exactly the same number and type of chromosome found in the mother cell.

The process is called mitosis, and all living cells (with the exception of bacteria and viruses, which have no chromosomes, and the egg and the sperm, which have a mechanism all their own) reproduce in this manner. From the beginning scientists suspected that the chromosomes were involved in heredity. With

Mendel's rediscovery their suspicions were confirmed. Chromosomes are the vehicles for Mendel's genes.

The number of chromosomes vary in different species. Mendel's sweet peas have 14, some flies have 8, mice 20, monkeys 42, crabs and lobsters as many as 500. You have 46. It is actually more accurate to think of yourself as having 23 pairs of chromosomes—one set from each parent.

There is an important exception to the rule that every cell in every species has the full complement of its allotted chromosomes. If the egg and the sperm each had 46 chromosomes at the time of fertilization, the fertilized egg (zygote) from which you develop would have 92 chromosomes. Your children would start life with 184 etc., etc.—clearly an impossibility. To prevent this monstrous accumulation, there is a special type of cell division specific for germ cells—meiosis. In preparation for fertilization, one cell division takes place without replication of the chromosomes—the cell now has 23.

The division is not consistent, however. If it were, one or more of your grandparents would be completely dealt out of your inheritance. Instead, there is a shuffling of chromosomes so that the egg and the sperm from which you were conceived have chromosomes from each of your maternal and paternal grandparents. The variety possible in such a shuffling allows for at least 8,000,000 different combinations in each offspring.

An additional mechanism provides even greater variety. A process known as crossing over provides new recombinations of parts of chromosomes. Now the possibilities for variety soar to many millions. It would be safe to say that except for identical twins, no 2 of the 40 billion humans that have lived have ever had exactly the same genetic endowment. Achieving variety in new individuals is what sexual reproduction (biologically) is all about. Even bacteria have sex—they exchange genetic material before dividing.

Actually the egg which has all the information to make a new individual (identical with the mother, of course) and the nourishment to start it growing can in some species be triggered to produce itself without a sperm (parthenogenesis). In the bee the unfertilized eggs produce only male bees, fertilized eggs produce female bees. There are colonies of lizards in which not a single male has been identified among hundreds of females. Yet the latter reproduce.

Still another form of reproduction bypassing not only the opposite sex but also the sex cells (egg and sperm) has been in the headlines in recent months. Cloning, also dubbed "wombs for rent," aims to give you a child that is an exact replica of one of your favorite people. All you need is one of the chosen individual's body cells. Because every cell in the body has a complete set of genes, it should be possible to put the nucleus of the cell into an egg whose own nucleus has been removed. Start the egg dividing, place it into a uterus of choice, and then wait the usual nine months for the new copy to develop.

If you have ever grown a plant from a cutting (no seed), you have achieved cloning. Can it be accomplished in higher forms of life? A few years ago a British embryologist made a start. He took the nucleus of an intestinal cell from a newly hatched tadpole and transplanted it into a frog's egg whose nucleus had been removed. About 4 percent developed into adult frogs. When he used nuclei from embryos, 30 percent became normal adults. Of course, using a cell of an embryo will not give you a preview of the finished product.

Can cloning be accomplished in humans? The prospect of mass producing identical persons is chilling to scientists and nonscientists as well. (To the gifted film creator of *Sleeper,* it is also hilarious.)

There are scientific as well as social and ethical problems. Obtaining a cell from the individual you choose is easy. Every time you brush your teeth you spit out many epithelial cells from the lining of your mouth. Each has a complete set of genes—a blueprint for a whole human being. The biggest problem in cloning is how to turn back the clock on the activity of the cell you choose. You start life with a single cell, and as the cell keeps dividing, the daughter cells differentiate into skin, liver, blood, etc. Each one retains its original assortment of genes, but once differentiated, only the genes required to maintain it as skin, liver, blood, etc. remain active. The other genes are still there but repressed. Can they be de-repressed? No one has yet tried.

Indications are that for the foreseeable future we shall continue to rely on sex and our sex cells for reproduction. How is sex determined? Of the twenty-three pairs of chromosomes in each of your cells, twenty-two (autosomes) are identical contributions from each of your parents. The twenty-third pair is the one that determines your sex. A male has a pair of unlike chromosomes—a large one called X inherited from his mother and a small chromosome called Y inherited from his father. The presence of the latter determines his male characteristics.

A female has two X chromosomes, one from her mother and one from her father. During meiosis, when the egg and the sperm are reduced to twenty-three chromosomes, the egg will always have an X to transmit. (It can be either her mother's or her father's X.) The sperm can end up with either an X (from his mother) or a Y (from his father). If the X-bearing sperm reaches and fertilizes the egg, the offspring with XX is female. If the Y-bearing sperm fertilizes the egg, the offspring is male. Researchers report progress in helping choose the sex of a baby by helping either the X or the Y sperm to get involved.

Because the X chromosome is large, it carries information for a large number of traits entirely unrelated to sex. More than seventy have been identified to date. A defect on the X chromosome will often not be harmful to the female because she has her other X chromosome to carry on for her. The male, however, with a defect on the X chromosome has no such protection. Hemophilia, color blindness, retinitis pigmentosa, and some forms of muscular dystrophy are among these sex-linked disorders. The woman is the carrier, the man the victim.

There was a time when it was suggested that females were biologically superior because of the two large X chromosomes. In the early 1960's, however, Dr. Mary Lyon found that actually only *one* X chromosome is functioning in each of a woman's cells. During fetal life, after development is complete, one X chromosome (chance determines which) stops working. If women are indeed biologically superior to men, it cannot be attributed to their extra X.

The role of chromosomes in disease came into its own in 1956, when scientists learned that the human cell has forty-six, not the forty-eight they had mistakenly counted in the past. It signaled the identification of a score of hereditary disorders where the chromosomes were either too few or too many, or where parts of chromosomes were either deleted or misplaced on other chromosomes. Only three years later an old and familiar disorder which had puzzled doctors for centuries was revealed to be due to an extra chromosome—Down's disease (mongolism, Chapter Three).

In 1970 cytogenetics (study of chromosomes) entered a new phase. Until then only the number, size, and shape could be identified. Now with new staining techniques it is possible for the first time to identify chemical differences in the chromosomes —perhaps even to locate individual genes. Today specific markers for specific genes have been identified on almost forty of the forty-six. Not only are new abnormalities being identified at an accelerated rate, but a new picture of normal variation is emerging as well.

Even with the new techniques chromosomes in most genetic disorders still add up to forty-six, each of which is a normal size and normal shape. The forty-six volumes need to have their pages cut to reveal their essential information. What are chromosomes made of? Even before chromosomes were discovered, a young

Swiss chemist, fresh from graduate school, isolated two sub-stances from the nuclei of cells: protein and a nonprotein fraction rich in phosphorus—DNA. Was it the protein or the DNA that held the secret of life?

Proteins make up more than half the body—skin, muscles, blood, hormones, and the enzymes that are the middlemen for all the chemical reactions in the body etc. Even in those days with biochemistry still in its infancy, the major importance of protein's very large molecules, made up of building blocks of many different amino acids, was undisputed. When DNA was subsequently analyzed, it turned out to be a relatively simple chemical—a molecule of sugar, a molecule of phosphate, and four molecules identified as adenine, guanine, cytosine, and thymine (later a substance similar to DNA but differing in minor respects, RNA, was also identified).

DNA, a substance with fewer ingredients than a modest dinner, seemed too simple to direct heredity. Friedrich Miescher clung to his faith in DNA, but like his contemporary Gregor Mendel, many years were to pass before he was proved right.

DNA faded into obscurity as the years went by. Chemists still hoped new evidence would emerge to identify the chemical responsible for heredity, and their guess was that it would turn out to be protein. In 1944 three Rockefeller University scientists who were investigating the transformation of a harmless Type 2 pneumococcus bacteria into a virulent lethal Type 3 announced that they had isolated and identified the chemical responsible for the transformation. It was DNA extracted from the dead cells of the Type 3 germ. DNA, not protein, carries hereditary instructions.

Dr. Oswald T. Avery and his associates made their momentous announcement rather modestly. They knew the significance of what they had found, but they also knew that there was no theoretical basis for how DNA with a monotonous repetition of four simple bases could carry out the complex tasks assigned to it.

(Supposedly when the Nobel committee considered them for a prize, the decision was "not yet." Avery died before he got that recognition, but scientists have since agreed that his contribution was historic.)

Further proof that DNA, not protein, is the hereditary substance came from experiments with viruses—organisms at the threshold of life. While every virus has its own genetic instructions and its own protein coat, it cannot make its protein by itself. It sustains itself by invading a living cell—bacteria, plant, animal, human—and taking over the cell's machinery. The cell now follows the genetic instructions of the virus and produces the protein the virus needs. When Drs. Alfred Hershey and Martha Chase allowed viruses to infect bacteria, they learned that only the DNA of the virus enters the cell, takes over, and reproduces itself. The protein remains outside.

Dr. Avery's announcement also spurred renewed interest in DNA among other scientists. The last objection to DNA was dispelled when Columbia University biochemist Dr. Erwin Chargaff discovered that the four bases are not a monotonous repetition of AGCTAGCTAGCT etc. but rather follow each other in an arbitrary order. The sequence is different in each living thing. Another of his discoveries was to be the key to the final solution of how DNA accomplishes its feat of replicating itself. The amount of adenine (A) is always equal to guanine (G), and cytosine (C) is always equal to thymine (T).

Suddenly the race was on for what would turn out to be one of the most important scientific discoveries of modern times—how DNA controls heredity, growth, health, disease, and even longevity.

By 1953 the facts were all there waiting to be put together. DNA is the chemical of heredity; the information is coded in the almost unending sequence of the nucleotides (a nucleotide is a molecule of sugar, a molecule of phosphate, and a base pair); X-ray pictures of DNA suggested that it is a helix—not unlike a spiral staircase. The last fact was not unexpected. The world-famous physical chemist Linus Pauling, who was also in the race, had recently discovered that the other vital molecules of life, proteins, are a triple helix.

It was all put together by a twenty-five-year-old ex-quiz kid from Chicago and a brilliant but still unrecognized British theoretical physicist. James Watson was twenty-three, with a PhD in biology, when he came to Cambridge University in 1951. His goal was to learn more about physics and chemistry so he could solve the problem of the gene. There he met Francis Crick, who had become interested in biology after wartime work including radar. He was one of the few scientists in the lab who shared Watson's enthusiasm for DNA.

They set about to build a model that would fit all the facts and could explain not only how the genetic information is stored in DNA, but also how it can replicate itself with speed and accuracy. They had the answer even before all the parts of their new model were delivered.

Nobel Laureate Dr. John Kendrew, in whose laboratory Dr. Watson worked briefly upon his arrival at Cambridge, described the event. "They looked at the new X ray photographs, they wondered about Chargaff's base pairing rules, they tried all sorts of models and the upshot was that in only a few weeks after one or two false starts, they actually solved the whole thing. . . . It is a good example of one of those intuitive jumps which happens in science from time to time. You may call it genius, you may call it inspiration. . . ." The scientific world called it momentous.

The Watson-Crick DNA is a double helix—two long fibers wound around each other like a spiral staircase, with a very long backbone made up of alternating molecules of sugar and phosphate. The rungs of the ladder are the four bases—AGCT. In order for the rungs to fill the spaces between the sides of the ladder properly, A must be paired with T and G with C. The bases are attached to each other with very weak chemical bonds (hydrogen) allowing them to be separated easily.

When the DNA is ready to make a copy of itself, the double helix unwinds into two separate single strands. A new strand forms alongside the single strand when an A picks up a T and a G picks up a C from the nucleotides lying loose in the cell. The two strands now form a new helix. There are two double helixes where there was formerly one. The cell is ready to divide into two daughter cells with identical information. The whole process functions with incredible efficiency.

It seemed almost too simple to be true! Could a chain of 200,000 nucleotides unwind in minutes without getting tangled, pick up a new partner, and wind itself into a double helix again? A couple of years later a young researcher at Washington University, Dr. Arthur Kornberg, made it happen in a test tube.

Thanks to Dr. Watson and Dr. Crick, the gene is no longer a concept. It is a concrete chemical entity—a sequence of nucleotides strung along a section of DNA. Each gene is a piece of heredity information. Scientists estimate that we have about 100,000 genes made up of 10 billion nucleotides. These are the numbers to ponder when you hear talk of creating life from chemicals on the shelf.

Precisely what does the gene do with its information so carefully replicated every time a new cell is made? The main function of the genes is to direct the production of proteins. The early biochemists were right when they identified proteins as the basic molecules of life. DNA is the blueprint.

We have enough information in our genes to code for 10,000,000 chains that will be assembled to make up our proteins. When you read about genes for blue or brown eyes, or proper utilization of milk, or proper metabolism of fats, the genes do not dictate the instructions directly. They direct the production of specific proteins—enzymes, the catalysts that make all chemical processes possible. So the gene for brown eyes dictates an enzyme that will in turn dictate the production of pigments that ultimately show up in your eyes. As many as ten enzymes may be required. Our total machinery keeps going with the help of thousands of enzymes.

The first link between genes and enzymes was made at the turn of the century by a British physician who discovered a curious condition among some of his patients—black urine. Sir Archibald Garrod suspected that the strange substance was a product of faulty metabolism owing to faulty enzymes. After studying the patients' families (there were siblings involved), he learned that although the children were affected, their parents were not. Another item of interest—the parents in all the families he studied were first cousins. When he discussed it with his friend, a leading geneticist, Dr. William Bateson immediately recognized that the pattern of the disease followed Mendel's laws. The children had inherited a defective recessive gene from each of their parents.

In the next few years Dr. Garrod identified three more diseases that fit the same pattern. With the publication of *Inborn Errors of Metabolism* in 1908, medical history was made. It took almost thirty years, however, for history to catch up with him. Like Mendel and Miescher, he was before his time. The concept that a gene controls an enzyme that in turn controls the metabolism of specific substances could not find a ready audience in his day. Physicians were not tuned in to genetics and biochemistry; geneticists were not concerned with human disease.

The one gene-one enzyme hypothesis became fact decades later when geneticists Drs. George Beadle and Edward Tatum proved it beyond a doubt in 1941. Their experiments with bread molds confirmed what Garrod had observed in humans: All biochemical activity is controlled by genes; every process is a series of steps; each step is controlled by a single gene.

Still to be explained was how the gene does its work. DNA sits in the nucleus of the cell like a top executive giving directions and controlling production without itself getting out into the factory. The assembly line is in the cytoplasm of the cell where the amino acids, the building blocks of protein, are floating around. Another nagging question was: How is the information in the four-letter alphabet of DNA transcribed to the twenty-letter alphabet of proteins (twenty amino acids are the building blocks of the protein chains. You can make about half the amino acids in your own cells. The other half you must take in already made by plants or other animals—hence the importance of including adequate and appropriate protein foods in your daily diet).

When the answers came in, nature again revealed an elegance and competence unrivaled by anything man has yet devised.

To fill an order for a specific protein, it is clearly not necessary for the entire DNA stretch to unwind and copy itself. Instead, only the portion with the required gene gets into action. It serves as a template for a substance very similar to DNA, called messenger RNA. (RNA differs slightly from DNA in its sugar molecule and in one of its bases—uracil instead of thymine.) The RNA leaves the nucleus with its message. In the cytoplasm it makes its way to another RNA-containing structure—the ribosome—where the actual assembly of the protein will take place. Still another RNA, transfer RNA, picks up the appropriate amino acids from those lying loose in the cell and brings them to the ribosome, where they are built up into chains according to the directions brought out of the nucleus by the m/RNA.

The final question was how could the DNA with only four bases at its disposal pick out the appropriate amino acids among the twenty that will ultimately be a protein molecule made up of hundreds of amino acids in a proper sequence? The scientific world got the answer at the Fifth International Biochemical Congress in Moscow in 1961. (The meeting was a first in more than one respect. It was the first large-scale contact between Russian biochemists and the molecular biologists of the rest of the world. Molecular biology had long been taboo in the Soviet Union, where it was labeled non-Marxian.)

Dr. Marshall Nirenberg, a young National Institutes of Health researcher, originally read his paper to a small audience. Probably no more than a few dozen of the 5,000 participants heard it. But when its importance was brought to Dr. Crick's attention, he immediately invited Dr. Nirenberg to repeat it at one of the prestigious symposia, in a large lecture hall with simultaneous translation into four languages. Dr. Nirenberg had cracked the genetic code—three nucleotides of DNA and RNA specify the particular amino acid the protein needs. He proved it in a test tube for a simple protein.

In contrast with the neglect suffered by some of the pioneers in genetics, Dr. Nirenberg received instant acclaim from his colleagues. In the next few years the codes for all the other amino acids were also worked out.

It was now possible to get down to a single molecule to track down mutations (mistakes in heredity). If a portion of a gene does not copy itself faithfully, the change will be passed down to every one of its descendant cells. A mistake in the DNA is repeated in the RNA. The code sends out a wrong message; the wrong amino acid occupies a space on a protein molecule where it does not belong. The enzyme or other protein is faulty; normal function is disrupted.

In rare instances the mutations are good; they may confer an advantage. This is how evolution came about. Sometimes the mutation is so serious as to be incompatible with life. Sometimes it can be so trivial that it is of no consequence. Each of us has six to ten defective genes and is none the worse for it.

It can also happen that the mistake will result in an individual who, like a car that comes off the assembly line with a defect in the steering mechanism, can function up to a point and then break down. So it is with the range of genetic diseases to which we are vulnerable.

If a good typist were to copy a book with all the information in our DNA, you could expect about one mistake in every 20 pages.

36

In nature the mistakes occur about once in every 10,000,000 pages. Rare as the mistakes are, they take a large toll in human life and well-being.

The following chapters will bring you up to date on what can now be done to diminish the mistakes and their consequences.

2

The New Look of Genetic Counseling— Tay-Sachs Disease: A Prototype

Until not too long ago when a parent of a child born with a genetic disorder asked, "Why did it happen, and can it happen again?" the usual answer was a large dose of sympathy and a mathematical guess about future recurrence. Indeed, the only way a family at risk could be assured of never bearing another affected child was to bear no children at all.

Today, thanks to new biochemical knowledge, new tools, and new techniques, an increasing number of such parents are now offered the option of bearing only children free of the disorder. Indeed so significant are the strides made in recent years that genetic counseling can now be viewed as the newest arrival in the arena of preventive medicine.

In contrast with the traditional lag between scientific discovery in the laboratory and clinical application in the doctor's office, new developments in genetics are sometimes implemented within months of their discovery. Such has been the case with Tay-Sachs disease.

Helen and Jack knew nothing of Tay-Sachs disease when they planned their first baby. "I think I had once seen it in print," she recalls, "but I doubt that I could have spelled it." Even if it had been familiar to them, they would probably not have given it a second thought. In their middle twenties, with no unusual illnesses in their own past or their families', they experienced no more than the occasional apprehension common to most expectant parents.

When Susan was born (without complications), she was all they had hoped for—healthy and beautiful. Her development in the next few months continued to fulfill their expectations. Helen began thinking of another baby; she wanted her family complete before she was thirty, and she knew she would have no problem extending her leave from her high school teaching job.

When the change started in Susan, it was so imperceptible that it was difficult to date it precisely. There was no doubt, however, that the changes were there and all for the worse. Objects that used to delight her no longer elicited a response. Now when she turned over, her arms flailed helplessly in a futile effort to turn back. Not only was she not progressing, but she was clearly deteriorating.

By the time she was eight months old Susan's condition was given a name: diagnosis, Tay-Sachs disease; prognosis, early death.

Not the least of the shock was the disclosure that Susan's illness was hereditary, that each of them had transmitted to her a defective gene of whose presence they were completely unaware. For the disease to manifest itself, the defective gene must be passed on in a double dose—one from each parent. The defective gene can be passed on in a single dose for generations, as must have happened in Helen's and Jack's families, with no recollection in either family of such an illness. (On the other hand, a look into the

40

past sometimes reveals that there indeed were such children born. They were often not properly identified and even less talked about.)

Susan's first birthday was marked with little joy. By this time she could barely sit up. Swallowing was difficult and her small food intake was only due to their perseverance and patience. On two occasions she suffered blackouts and convulsions.

What could they look forward to with a second pregnancy? Could their luck be just as bad the second time around?

But this time they did not have to rely on luck. While there is still no treatment for Susan, there are now discoveries that make it possible to predict with almost 100 percent certainty if the unborn baby is affected, to terminate the pregnancy with safety if such is the decision of the parents and the doctor, to monitor future pregnancies and to say with assurance when a baby free of the disease is being carried, and to identify and warn other parents at risk without waiting for the first tragedy to occur.

The story begins many centuries ago in an area of Eastern Europe straddling the Polish-Russian border. Here in the small Jewish towns isolated from the mainstream of the land in which they lived, a small number of families must have suffered the grim tragedy of watching a normal healthy baby begin to deteriorate into a blind, paralyzed, vegetablelike existence. Curiously enough, virtually nothing about it was recorded until the occupants of this area began a mass migration to the United States and Western Europe in the nineteenth century. By 1880 an English eye doctor, Warren Tay, found the cherry red spot on the retina that accounts for the blindness, and in 1887 the neurologist Dr. Bernard Sachs described the rest of the syndrome.

Helen and Jack are among the 6,000,000 Jews in the United States who are descendants of those Russian-Polish migrants. They are also among the one in thirty who are carriers of the recessive gene responsible for Tay-Sachs disease. A survey of the grandparents of Tay-Sachs infants in the New York area revealed

41

that the majority came from a territory that includes most of northeastern Poland, southern Lithuania, and an adjacent section of Byelorussia.

Further proof of its origin comes from Israel, where among its 3,000,000 Jews, Tay-Sachs disease is virtually unknown among the immigrants from Asia and North Africa (Sephardic) and, as in the rest of the world, is limited almost exclusively to those of Eastern European descent. (While it has been found in non-Jews as well, the European Jews account for at least 85 percent of all cases.)

It has been known for many years that the problem in Tay-Sachs disease is an abnormal accumulation of fatty substances (gangliosides) in the brain and other parts of the nervous system. The search for the missing enzyme responsible for splitting these fats was pursued in a number of different laboratories. Attention finally narrowed down to a specific chemical area, that of hexosaminidase activity. Scientists were frustrated, however, in nailing down hexosaminidase deficiency as the culprit when it was learned that Tay-Sachs babies not only did not suffer from a deficiency but on the contrary sometimes had elevated levels.

It was not until 1969 that two researchers at the University of California School of Medicine, San Diego, dispelled the mystery. Hexosaminidase is present in two components—A and B. While the normal individual has mostly hex-A in his blood, he has only traces of hex-B. The Tay-Sachs baby, on the other hand, is virtually lacking in hex-A. The trouble starts with the gene that dictates the instructions for the enzyme hex-A. No hex-A—no breakdown of the harmful fats.

When Drs. Shintaro Okada and John S. O'Brien published their findings in *Science* in August, 1969, they predicted that the immediate practical importance of their discovery was that the diseased Tay-Sachs baby could now be clearly identified when the symptoms appear. Taking it one step further, they also anticipated that the new knowledge could identify the disease in the unborn fetus when it was already known that the risk for a Tay-Sachs baby existed.

That prophecy was not long in being fulfilled, and it was no surprise that the first application took place at an institution which more than any in the world had been identified with concern and care for the victims of Tay-Sachs disease and their anguished parents, the Kingsbrook Jewish Medical Center in Brooklyn, New York. A few months after the report in *Science,* Dr. Bruno Volk (who had established the nation's first Tay-Sachs ward in 1953) and pediatric neurologist Dr. Larry Schneck, also long involved in the problem, met with a mother who had already lost a child to Tay-Sachs disease and who was now pregnant again.

"What we can now offer you is still experimental," Dr. Schneck explained, "but we think that it may be possible to find out if the child you are now carrying is free of the disease or endangered by it. The choice will then be yours as to whether you will continue the pregnancy or interrupt it."

Her response was one that dozens of young mothers were to make in the next few years: "Go ahead."

The process that would yield the hitherto-unavailable secrets of the fetus is known as amniocentesis, in which a sample of the fluid in which the fetus is suspended in the uterus is withdrawn from the mother's abdomen and studied. As far back as a century ago doctors were removing amniotic fluid in rare circumstances when they feared that too much was accumulating.

In 1952 British obstetrician Dr. Douglas Bevis pioneered the use of amniocentesis for diagnostic purposes. He withdrew a small sample of amniotic fluid to check the severity of blood destruction suffered by an Rh baby (see Chapter 5). In the next few years repeated use of amniocentesis with apparent safety to both mother and child suggested the enormous promise that this technique might hold for other hereditary disease.

Because the fetus sheds some of its own cells and products into the amniotic fluid as it develops, the fluid provides dozens of clues about the fetus' condition. Familiar laboratory techniques detect biochemical changes. Most exciting, however, are the new vistas opened up when scientists learned to grow human cells in culture, as they have been doing with bacteria for decades. Now, instead of depending on the limited number of cells present in the amniotic fluid, they can harvest millions of direct descendants of these cells in a matter of days.

For the dream of prenatal diagnosis to become a reality, two conditions had to be met: a precise test to identify the disorder and the ability to detect it in the amniotic fluid. With the discovery of hex-A deficiency in Tay-Sachs, the first condition was met. Only the future had the answer to the second.

To perform the amniocentesis, Drs. Schneck and Volk enlisted the services of an obstetrician who had by then had considerable experience with the procedure at Brooklyn's Downstate Medical Center—Dr. Carlo Valenti. Removing the amniotic fluid was a routine procedure for him, but then the suspense began to build. The first test revealed no hex-A—another Tay-Sachs baby. However, this was a first; they had to be sure. Maybe hex-A would still be produced if they waited. Two weeks later another amniocentesis was performed. The bad news was confirmed—still no hex-A. This baby would, like the other babies ending their lives in the ward upstairs, show no evidence of the disease at birth, but would within the first year of life follow the same inexorable course to death.

When the shock of the news wore off, the parents' decision was clear-cut—a therapeutic abortion. Examination of the fetus confirmed what the earlier tests had indicated—another Tay-Sachs baby. For the first time in centuries the birth of a Tay-Sachs baby was prevented!

Within the next year fourteen more couples who had already had one Tay-Sachs child came to Kingsbrook and asked that this time the pregnancy be monitored. Ten were given the good news that the baby would be free of the disease. The other four were not so lucky. All four chose abortion.

Among the fourteen couples were Helen and Jack. "We have done only a few cases," they were told, "but we think that we are on the right track." By now they were fully aware that there was no longer any hope for Susan, but if there was any for the future, they wanted that chance.

"I shall never forget the Thursday morning I received the preliminary report—it looks as if the baby is OK, but we want to wait two or three weeks for all the tests to be complete." Helen smiled as she continued. "We were jubilant, but one piece of news we kept to ourselves until David was born." Because Helen knew that it was possible to learn the baby's sex from the amniotic fluid, she asked if it could be determined as an "extra bonus." So that while they shared the good news with their anxious parents that this baby would be free of Tay-Sachs disease, only they and the doctor knew that it would be a boy.

When a genetic disease appears in a family for the first time, the question "Can it happen to us?" now becomes relevant for brothers and sisters, cousins, etc. Since both Helen and Jack have inherited the defective trait from *their* parents, there is a strong possibility that other members of the family have as well.

In the August, 1969, *Science* report, Drs. Okado and O'Brien included another significant discovery. Parents of Tay-Sachs children have a blood level of hex-A about halfway between that of an affected child and a normal individual. The one good gene each carries provides enough enzyme for their needs. They are healthy carriers. That they also have a defective gene was learned only when (purely by chance) they each transmitted it to the baby. With a relatively simple blood test it is now possible to identify a carrier before a baby is conceived. All children of carriers will not necessarily be carriers themselves. Now the sister or brother who is *not* a carrier can learn that they and their descendants need not fear the disease.

Helen and Jack wasted no time in urging their brothers and sisters to volunteer for the test. It took only a small volume of blood and a modest fee to the laboratory for Helen's recently married younger sister and her husband to learn that neither is a carrier. Jack's brother, already the father of two normal children, was resistant when the idea of being tested was first proposed. "It doesn't really matter," he argued, "we don't plan any future children, so why bother? And as far as our children are concerned, they can decide for themselves when they are older if they want to be tested." When it was pointed out to him that if a test now revealed that neither he nor his wife is a carrier, his children would be relieved of an unnecessary anxiety in their early adulthood, he had second thoughts about the test.

At risk for Tay-Sachs disease are not only relatives of known cases. With one in thirty Jews in the United States suspected of being carriers, that entire population is a risk.

The first large-scale search for carriers in a high-risk population was launched in 1971 by Johns Hopkins pediatrician Dr. Michael Kaback with the sponsorship of the John F. Kennedy Foundation. The goal was to reach 60,000 Jewish couples of childbearing age in the Washington-Baltimore area in the next two years. Many had never heard of the disease. Few were aware of the threat it might hold for them. Perhaps 150 to 200 were in danger of bearing a defective child.

Pleas from pulpits in area synagogues, as well as efforts by more than 100 community organizations, brought out several thousand for testing in the first few months. Among them were nine couples who all learned that they were carriers married to carriers. To date none had had a Tay-Sachs child. So far they had transmitted only the good gene. But they did learn that with every future pregnancy a one in four risk existed for an affected baby. In 1972 one of these couples learned from amniocentesis that the wife was carrying a Tay-Sachs baby. The interruption of that pregnancy marked the first time that the tragedy of a Tay-Sachs birth was prevented in a family alerted only by the screening program.

Dr. Kaback has since moved to Harbor General Hospital, University of California School of Medicine at Los Angeles, where more than half a million Jews can profit from the enthusiasm and know-how he brings to this problem.

Similar screening programs are being developed in other cities, including Philadelphia and Boston. Inquiries about setting up such programs continue to pour into the offices of the National Tay-Sachs and Allied Disease Foundation, New York City, from cities across the nation. In recent months several thousand college students in the New York area have been screened.

The new look of genetic counseling includes another new dimension—restoring and maintaining the emotional and psychological well-being of young people who have until now viewed themselves as normal (as they are, of course) and suddenly learn they are different. Some react with guilt, others with anger and denial. Some are just overwhelmed with the enormity of the burden that faces them.

"At first the family of a Tay-Sachs baby is too shocked to be overwhelmed with facts," says Mrs. Frances Berkwits, social worker at Kingsbrook's Tay-Sachs center. "Our first responsibility is to sustain them emotionally. Most parents want to keep their baby at home as long as possible. This enables them to come to grips with the hospitalization that is almost inevitable."

If there is a healthy child at home, Mrs. Berkwits helps keep his needs in perspective as well. And only when the parents are ready to think of the future does she discuss what the options are.

Sylvia and Jerry's first child was conceived with the help of a fertility drug. "Judy was worth waiting for" was the early consensus. But symptoms of Tay-Sachs first appeared when she was nine months old, and by her first birthday the diagnosis was made and confirmed. By her second birthday she had deteriorated to a state where hospitalization could no longer be avoided.

"The empty crib," Sylvia explains, "seemed to cry out to be occupied." Now they were ready for what Mrs. Berkwits had to tell them. When they were told about amniocentesis, it was no longer necessary to warn that it was still experimental for Tay-Sachs. Fortified with the knowledge that no matter what the outcome of the amniocentesis was, "we would never have to visit another child waiting to die in the hospital," Sylvia became pregnant again. This time it was without the help of a fertility drug.

She did not need a reminder to show up for the amniocentesis. After the most suspenseful weeks in their married life they learned that it was another Tay-Sachs baby. The decision was to abort. "We had no regrets about the abortion," says Sylvia, "only sorrow." And with the sorrow—depression. This is another period when the guidance of a professional other than the genetic counselor is needed and welcomed. Sylvia is now back at her job as a graphic artist, waiting eagerly to leave when the hoped-for new pregnancy is a reality.

There is no standard formula for successful genetic counseling for the wide range of situations encountered. There is, however, unanimous agreement that the first step is correct diagnosis—not always to be taken for granted in rare diseases, unfamiliar to the practicing physician. Correct and early diagnosis is especially important when the genetic disorder is one of the fifty that can now be treated with diet. For example, prompt action in galactosemia and PKU (Chapter 11) can mean the difference between a normal and a hopelessly retarded child.

Many of the tests can be performed only in specialized laboratories geared to perform rare and sophisticated procedures. Such services are now available nationwide. Fortunately both blood and amniotic fluid remain suitable for testing until arrival at the appropriate facility.

When there is good reason to believe that the disease is indeed hereditary, the question then is "How is it transmitted?"—through one parent (dominant) or both parents (recessive)—or does it fall into the category of sex-linked disorders usually transmitted by mothers to their sons?

48

To complete the picture, the genetic counselor will want to know the story of close and perhaps not so close relatives. (Counseling is of special importance in small communities where there has been much intermarriage.) And in diseases such as Huntington's disease where there are no biochemical markers or chromosomal abnormalities, a good family history may well be the only clue.

Some disorders that are apparent at birth may not be genetic at all; they may be the consequences of harmful drugs used by the mother during pregnancy or an infection which may have been trivial for her but devastating for the baby. (The early victims of thalidomide were suspected to be genetic, as were many babies born to mothers who had had German measles in the early months of pregnancy.)

Special vigilance is required for the baby who seems normal at birth but who is in fact suffering from a delayed-action "time bomb" with a disease that may show up months or even years later. So it is not only with Tay-Sachs, but with other diseases whose stories appear in detail in later chapters—sickle cell, thalassemia, Wilson's, and Huntington's.

Sometimes a disorder that has long been labeled "genetic" turns out not to be that at all when more is learned about it. Such is the case of a rare disease called kuru, believed to be genetic because it ran in families but which has recently been attributed to a virus with long-delayed action.

Tay-Sachs is one of more than 100 disorders with a known enzyme or protein abnormality. Almost sixty can now be diagnosed in utero with amniocentesis, but by far the greatest use of amniocentesis for genetic counseling is not in the search of a single aberrant gene but for an abnormal chromosome—the repository of tens of thousands of genes. Leading the list is Down's syndrome (mongolism) which accounts for 95 percent of all amniocentesis, and whose story merits its own chapter.

It has been estimated that 1 in 500 couples can benefit from genetic counseling. How many of them are receiving it? How well do they understand what they are getting? What do they do with the information they get?

To date reports have been largely anecdotal. The first large-scale study covering a period of years was reported by Dr. Cedric O. Carter, director of the Clinical Genetics Unit at the Institute of Child Health in London. (Britain established its first genetic clinic in 1946 under the leadership of Dr. J. A. Fraser Roberts, co-author with Dr. Carter of the report on the study in *The Lancet,* February, 1971.)

Among those counseled were 455 couples, all with at least one affected child and who had specifically sought advice on the risk of future recurrence. They were followed up three to ten years after the counseling. Dr. Carter and his colleagues found that "on the whole the parents had understood the information they were given." Moreover, they made "responsible decisions" on the basis of this information. Where the risk of recurrence was high, two-thirds were deterred from planning future children and took steps that included adoption, contraception, sterilization, and, in some instances artificial insemination (at their own and not the counselor's suggestion).

Even among the low risk, almost one-quarter were deterred from future pregnancy. How a parent views a risk does not always coincide with the genetic counselor. One mother when told that the odds for a recurrence of her child's abnormality was one in twenty-five remarked that to her it was one in two, either the next child would be healthy or it would be affected. *Her* decision was to adopt.

Subsequent reports support Dr. Carter's findings to some extent while others relate a less optimistic story. While still a medical student, Dr. Claire O. Leonard of Johns Hopkins University School of Medicine interviewed 77 families who had been counseled following the birth of a baby with a genetic disorder. Unlike Dr. Carter's families, who for the most part showed a good understanding of the information they had received, fewer than half of Dr. Leonard's group retained information that could be viewed as useful to them. One-quarter had faulty memories of the information, and the comprehension of one-quarter was so garbled that the information was virtually useless. Some gave correct answers during the interview but really did not understand what they were saying. It was almost as if they wanted to score a high mark on a test.

Some families went to great lengths to *deny* the facts. One family insisted that cystic fibrosis has a good prognosis; two mothers would not allow amniocentesis on their daughters; one family clearly stuck to the belief that the disease in question was not genetic, and another refused to permit tests on other children in the family; one father denied paternity!

A very significant outcome of Dr. Leonard's study was the disclosure that the burden of the disease, rather than the risk of recurrence, was more critical in making parents think twice about future childbearing. So Down's syndrome, with a small chance of recurrence but a lifetime burden, poses more of a threat than PKU with a one in four risk but amenable to treatment.

There were other differences between the two groups. Dr. Carter's patients were all motivated; they initiated the counseling themselves. A large proportion were well educated and from upper socioeconomic groups. All had been counseled by either Dr. Carter or Dr. Fraser personally. By contrast, Dr. Leonard's group had been *sent* for counseling, were more limited in their educational backgrounds, and had received their counseling from a variety of professional individuals. In some instances they were confused when doctors gave them the facts and then left them to make their own decisions; they were accustomed to look to their doctor for more forthright advice.

What are the prospects for better acceptance of genetic counseling not only by those who need it today but also by the young people who in the not too distant future will be the parents of tomorrow?

One answer comes from an event that took place on December

29, 1972, in Washington, D. C., at the 139th Annual Meeting of the American Association for Advancement of Science. A full-day symposium, "Genetics and Man" brought together hundreds of scientists and young people under the joint sponsorship of the Youth Council of the AAAS and the Task Force on Genetics and Reproduction at Yale University.

Discussed that day were both the scientific and social aspects of the "new genetics." The interaction between the prestigious panel of experts and the large number of young men and women participants raised great hopes that the coming generation will bring to the problem greater knowledge and, it is hoped, greater responsiveness.

"You cannot choose your children's genes," Dr. Y. Edward Hsia, associate professor of human genetics, pediatrics, and medicine at Yale, told the symposium, "but you may be forewarned against a major disease without a child being born. And when the risk is negligible, go ahead."

A program now in progress at Yale promises to accomplish exactly that and to avert some of the pitfalls that genetic counseling often encounters. A family usually arrives at the Yale clinic, after the birth of an affected child and at the suggestion of the doctor. Many are bewildered about the services that are about to be offered to them. "Why are we here? Did we do something wrong to contribute to our child's condition? What can you do for us? How much will it cost?"

To answer these questions, the Yale program provides the services of a team of professionals and a continuity that is designed to meet the specific needs of each family. The first member of the team they meet is a specially trained nurse-coordinator who obtains whatever data are already available. The physician then looks it over. Sometimes he may decide he wants more details or more tests. Since most families are not yet ready for a lecture on science and math, the social worker now becomes involved.

By the time the family is ready for the next step—the current situation and the options for tomorrow—they approach it with the assurance that someone has taken heed of their problems. In fact, the social worker participates in the counseling session with the physician. Alert to the reactions of the family, it is often the social worker who helps pose appropriate questions.

No one at this point expects that the information given now will be completely absorbed and retained. To reinforce it, a letter summarizing the contents of the conference is sent out a few weeks later. The family now have a permanent record to which they can refer. Their personal physician also receives a copy of the report.

Several months later another letter is sent inquiring, "Did you understand what we are trying to tell you? Were you satisfied? Did you act on the information? Was it worthwhile?"

Of the seventy-three families followed up, seventy-two replied. Only one, found to have no genetic disease, discarded the inquiry.

One father of a Down's syndrome child assessed the worth as follows, "I would have paid ten times the cost if it had been offered to me a few years back."

The overall results at the Yale clinic so far are a little less clear-cut than Dr. Carter's but not as discouraging as Dr. Leonard's. Among the high-risk group the majority indicated that they would now have second thoughts about future pregnancies, but a few became pregnant nevertheless. A few rejected, a few denied, and a few forgot what they had been told.

"It is a plus," says Dr. Hsia, "if the parents get no more than a better understanding of the nature of their child's illness—even if their plans for future children are unchanged."

If a gap exists between what genetic counseling has to offer and what currently is being accepted, it has not succeeded in disheartening professionals in the field. Writing in *Medical World News,* Dr. Betty Danes, Cornell University School of Medicine, reminds her physician readers that "after years of explosive growth, genetic counseling is approaching its infancy."

All indications are that the baby is robust and is growing well. New hope is here for before-the-fact counseling, thanks to tests that can identify carriers of more than seventy disorders. In disorders where amniocentesis provides no clues to abnormalities, scientists now use other techniques to visualize the fetus—such as ultrasound to identify structural defects.

Dr. Valenti is hard at work perfecting an instrument that will make it possible to view the fetus directly. It is hoped that in the not too distant future it will also be possible to obtain blood and other specimens for study from the fetus itself.

In at least one disorder for which no predictive tests are available, scientists have found that the defective gene is closely linked to another trait (harmless) that *can* be identified. Dystrophia myotonica incapacitates both mentally and physically, though it may not strike until the victims are adults and parents. The clue is a gene that is responsible for the secretion of a substance in the saliva that has absolutely nothing to do with the disease. The sole link is that the two genes are close neighbors on the same chromosome and are transmitted together.

Not only can the "secretor" gene be found in carriers, but it has recently been learned that it can be detected as early as the ninth week of pregnancy in the developing fetus. This example of "guilt by association" is another instance of the ingenuity researchers are applying to nagging problems. It may well open the way to similar discoveries in disorders like Huntington's disease where no such help now exists.

Laboratory and counseling services have proliferated in recent years. A generation ago there were scarcely a couple of dozen such facilities in the entire country. In 1968, when the National Foundation-March of Dimes published the first edition of the *International Directory of Genetic Services* compiled by Dr. Henry T. Lynch, Creighton University School of Medicine, 156 services were listed. By 1974 the directory listed 890 scientists and centers for counseling services, including 251 offering amniocentesis.

The New Look of Genetic Counseling—Tay-Sachs Disease

With the growth of genetic counseling new questions have arisen on who should do the counseling: a geneticist; a physician trained in genetics; a graduate of short-term counseling course; individuals trained for a specific disorder and its unique burden; a team such as Yale offers? So far the experiences have been both good and not so good with all categories. The final answer is by no means in.

The January, 1973, landmark decision by the U.S. Supreme Court striking down prohibition of abortion in all fifty states now removes legal restraints that may have been a barrier in the past. Moreover where religious beliefs have been a barrier to both contraception and abortion, they too are being changed when the family is faced with the reality of the situation.

Perhaps the largest contribution genetic counseling can make is the reassurance to the large proportion of families counseled where the answer is "It is OK—go ahead." Convincing evidence to that effect was presented to the symposium by Dr. Kaback. A review of 1,500 amniocenteses revealed that almost *1,400* were normal. For the 110 that were not, the parents all had the option of interrupting the pregnancy.

Back in 1955 the renowned Columbia University Professor Franz Kallman told the American Society of Human Genetics of a plea by one of his anxious patients, "We want hope—not just statistics."

Helen and Jack, Sylvia and Jerry, and thousands of others can tell you that is exactly what genetic counseling has given them.

3

Down's Syndrome—Mongolism

Steven is not the only four-year-old on his block picked up for nursery school in the morning. He is, however, the only one to be dropped off at a program that would have stirred skepticism in the not too distant past, for he is among 6,000 children born in the United States every year with Down's syndrome, commonly known as mongolism.

While Steven will do better at nursery school than many of the other mentally retarded children and will, it is hoped, move up into a regular school program in time, he will probably reach a mental plateau at the age of eight or nine into which he may well be locked for the rest of his life.

Counseling with Down's syndrome often starts not with the genetic counselor but with the doctor in the hospital who breaks the news to the family that they will be taking home a baby quite different from the one they had envisioned and prepared for. How he tells them may well set the tone for how they will cope. They see before them possibly decades of a crushing emotional and financial burden.

As a matter of fact, Steven's parents, who had a normal two-year-old as well, were unable to accept him at the beginning and arranged for him to be cared for in a foster home. By the time he was two months old the pull to bring him back to the family prevailed—a decision they have had no reason to regret. They are learning that the warmth and understanding he derives from a close family relationship in his early years are the best insurance that he can develop to his fullest potential, limited as that might be.

Also in their future, however, is the promise that they need never again bear another child with the disorder. Genetic counseling now enables a family at risk to be reassured in a future pregnancy when the fetus is free of the abnormality and to interrupt the pregnancy if the fetus is affected. Amniocentesis, the process of withdrawing a sample of the fluid surrounding the fetus in the womb during the fifteenth to sixteenth week of its development and studying the cells it sheds, tells the story (see Chapter 2). Indeed, more than 90 percent of all amniocenteses are performed in the search for Down's syndrome.

Unlike Tay-Sachs disease, sickle cell disease, thalassemia, and other disorders, identification of Down's syndrome is usually made within the first few weeks of life. The slanting eyes, flat facial profile, lower than normal ears, short, broad hands, curved little finger, wide space between the toes, telltale simian crease across the palm, and most significant of all, the very slow reflex responses add up to a portent of the mental retardation and physical makeup that will characterize the child's life and development.

It was first recognized as a distinct disorder in 1866 by a British physician, Dr. Langdon Down, whose name it now bears. Because it was his impression that victims bore some resemblance to Orientals, he described them as "mongoloid"—a misnomer that has persisted for a century and is still familiar to the general public. There is a special irony in Dr. Down's labeling a disease associated with subnormal development and mental retardation with a particular ethnic group, for he was clearly not a racist. On the contrary, he espoused a strong belief in the unity of mankind and attacked apologists of slavery in America.

Despite the "mongoloid" label, we have since learned that the syndrome can be readily recognized in all racial grops, including Eskimos, Seminole Indians, blacks, and Orientals. Some Japanese doctors have observed that to them Down's syndrome patients look "strikingly European." No matter what his origin, the individual with Down's syndrome has the ethnic look of his own group and a characteristic Down's look as well.

The overall incidence of Down's syndrome has been estimated as 1 in 600 live births. (A more precise figure might be 1 in 457 obtained by Dr. Jacob Wahrman of Hebrew University, who studied all live births in a section of Jerusalem during a four-year period.) Among mothers from eighteen to twenty the incidence is a low 1 in 2,300. It rises slowly to the age of thirty when it is 1 in 600, but after thirty-five the rise is very sharp, and it is most hazardous to women over forty.

There is evidence that this syndrome has affected mankind for more than 1,000 years but it is only since 1959 that a startling discovery revolutionized the thinking about it. It has long been known that the mother's age played a big role in its incidence. More than half of all such babies are born to mothers over thirty-five. Many additional theories were suggested; malfunctioning thyroid, adrenal or pituitary glands, tuberculosis and other infections, even alcoholism.

In 1959, only three years after the discovery that the normal human cell contains forty-six chromosomes, Dr. J. Lejeune and his colleagues at the University of Paris discovered that the victim of Down's syndrome has *forty-seven*. With Down's therefore a specific gene is not at fault and therefore the biochemical consequences cannot be tracked down in the same way they can be with diseases like G6PD deficiency, Tay-Sachs, sickle cell. What happens however when a whole chromosome, the repository of thousands of genes, is at fault?

Often it is incompatible with life. About one-third of all early spontaneous abortions are associated with chromosomal abnormalities. When the pregnancy is carried through successfully despite the chromosomal defect, the children exhibit a variety of effects ranging from trivial to severely impaired. Sometimes they can live to fifty or sixty handicapped both mentally and physically.

Such is the case with Down's syndrome, in which the extra chromosome disrupts a wide range of vital functions.

In the past, many died early in life from infections to which they were excessively vulnerable. Modern antibiotics have minimized much of that hazard. In the absence of other gross physical handicaps, development can be relatively good especially at the beginning.

Such was the case with Steven who sat, walked, and used his hands not much slower than his older normal sister. It was only later when more intellectual skills were needed that progress began to lag and it was increasingly clear that he could never catch up or keep up.

Progress with some children has been so encouraging that some parents can easily be lulled into hopes that are unlikely to be fulfilled. "Debbie was admitted to public school only after a persistent effort on our part," reports her mother, a soft-spoken but determined woman of forty. Even the school professionals who initially resisted frankly acknowledge their surprise and pleasure at Debbie's accomplishments. She just celebrated her eighth birthday and helping her celebrate were four boys and girls from her class—an average second grade in the neighborhood elementary school.

Although she cannot keep up with them in all respects, she

enjoys reading, performs reasonably well in her after-school dancing class, and follows her favorite programs on TV with genuine pleasure and understanding. Her development to date is not only an indication of her own potential but also a reflection of the love and attention showered on her by her parents and two older sisters, both in college today.

How long she can continue in a regular classroom has not yet been determined. Indeed the increased life expectancy in Down's syndrome is fraught with many uncertainties for children like Steven and Debbie. No more than 20 percent survive after thirty, 8 percent after forty, and about 2.5 percent after fifty. And an increasing number will survive their parents.

"With an increase in life span," Dr. G. A. Jervis, Institute for Basic Research in Mental Retardation, New York, told a New York Academy of Sciences Conference on Down's syndrome in November, 1969, "it has become more apparent that patients with Down's syndrome age prematurely." While deterioration in IQ or intellectual capacity is hard to measure, behavior and emotional changes are easily recognized—"from cheerfulness to sullenness, from playfulness to apathy, from docility to aggressiveness . . . speech is often lost . . . changes in personal habits such as incontinence and slovenliness in a habitually tidy patient."

Dr. Jervis had reported on evidence of "premature senility" in the brains of adults with Down's syndrome as far back as 1948. Since then additional confirmation has been presented by both him and other scientists. Among twenty-three who were between thirty-four and sixty-five at time of death (only five were over sixty), all showed unmistakable evidence of pathological changes in the brain characteristic of advanced senility.

Many families who were learning to cope with the present and mustering strength for a difficult future were at the same time living with an anxiety that it could happen again. Dr. Lejeune's discovery of the extra chromosome now made possible the positive identification of every victim. Was it possible to detect the

HEREDITY AND YOU

defect in the fetus as well? Fortunately this was the decade (the sixties) when rapid strides were being made in genetics—greater safety and skill in the techniques of amniocentesis, progress in the study of fetal cells, and an intensified look at the chromosomes themselves, both normal and abnormal.

Where does the forty-seventh chromosome come from? When an egg and a sperm cell matures, the forty-six chromosomes originally present are halved to twenty-three. Now when fertilization takes place the new cell (zygote) destined to become a new individual, will have the normal forty-six—twenty-three from each parent. Sometimes one set of chromosomes fails to separate—nondisjunction. The result is a sex cell with twenty-four chromosomes, which, when united with another cell with a normal twenty-three, adds up to forty-seven. The chromosome involved in the nondisjunction in Down's syndrome is No. 21. The baby has three No. 21 chromosomes, hence the term often used by scientists—trisomy No. 21. This phenomenon accounts for more than 95 percent of all Down's syndrome individuals. Nondisjunction appears to occur more often in the egg cells of older women; hence the greater danger of Down's syndrome in mothers over thirty-five.*

In 1960, a year after Dr. Lejeune's pioneering discovery of trisomy No. 21, another type of chromosomal abnormality and Down's syndrome was found, clinically identical with trisomy No. 21 but with a different basis for the chromosome defect. A portion of the No. 21 chromosome gets on to No. 14 or No. 15. The individual with such an abnormality appears normal in all respects since he has the usual amount of chromosomal material albeit some of it is in an unexpected location. He or she is a carrier of a "balanced translocation" and, like carriers of all defects, runs the risk of transmitting it to each of their offspring. When a child

* A small number of Down's syndrome cases are described as "mosaic" because they have a mixture of cells—some with the normal forty-six chromosomes and some with the abnormal forty-seven.

of a carrier inherits the abnormal chromosome and then receives a normal set of chromosomes from the other parent, he has inherited an excess amount of chromosomal material. Down's syndrome is the consequence.

Translocation trisomies can occur at any age and can be transmitted by the father as well as the mother. Because the risk of recurrence is very high (one in six if the mother is the carrier and one in ten through the father) and because, like other carrier defects, it can be found in other relatives, the identification of one member signals an urgent search for translocations among other members of the family. Fortunately translocations are rare, accounting for fewer than 3 percent of all of Down's syndrome victims.

The discovery of the chromosome abnormality gave impetus to the idea of looking for the defect in the fetus when there was reason to suspect the possibility of Down's syndrome. One of the earliest reports came from Dr. Carlo Valenti (who was to be the first to perform an amniocentesis for Tay-Sachs disease) and his colleagues, Dr. Edward J. Schutta and Tehila Keharty, at Brooklyn's Downstate Medical Center. It told the story of a translocation which was passed down for successive generations, silent and unsuspected and then manifested itself repeatedly in one young mother. In April, 1968, Dr. Valenti was consulted by a twenty-nine-year-old woman whose first pregnancy had ended in a spontaneous abortion. A year later she gave birth to a normal little girl. So far she had no reason to fear another pregnancy. Spontaneous abortions are not that rare, and there was no inkling of hereditary disease in the family. Two years later her first son was born—diagnosis Down's syndrome—and dead at five months. By this time she had learned of prenatal diagnosis and how she might be spared another tragedy.

The amniocentesis performed by Dr. Valenti did indeed spare her another tragedy; it was again a Down's syndrome. The decision was to interrupt the pregnancy and monitor the next.

63

A look back into the family history disclosed that she inherited a balanced translocation from her mother as did her brother. Her grandmother is normal, but her grandfather was identified as the carrier. To complete the pedigree, her normal little girl was tested. She too is a carrier and will of course be made aware of it when she is old enough to contemplate raising a family of her own.

At about the same time, nationally renowned geneticist Dr. Henry Nadler was scoring an even more dramatic triumph over Down's disease for a thirty-eight-year-old woman eager to start a family. She was fearful because her mother had borne three children with Down's syndrome. Examination of her chromosomes revealed that she was a translocation carrier. To that risk was added that posed by her age.

Nevertheless, fortified by the knowledge that her pregnancy could be monitored, she became pregnant only to learn that the fetus was affected. She chose to interrupt the pregnancy and within three months was pregnant again. This time amniocentesis revealed a girl with the normal complement of chromosomes. At forty-three she completed her family—again after amniocentesis revealed a normal boy.

"Here is a woman at almost *maximum risk,*" Dr. Nadler told a symposium on the Scientific and Ethical Considerations of Early Diagnosis of Human Genetic Defects, "who is able to have children but to select those children without chromosomal abnormalities."

There are at least 6,000,000 mentally retarded Americans today. The chromosome abnormality of Down's syndrome is only 1 among 100 causes. It is also one of the few which need not create a tragedy as the knowledge is here to prevent such births in high-risk women. While some would not accept the solution of amniocentesis and abortion, many more would if they were informed and if the services were made available to them.

One such program has been functioning on the north shore of Long Island since 1962. For many the route to genetic counseling is through the Nassau County Chapter of the Association for Help of Retarded Children (AHRC), Brookville, New York. "By the time the parents come to us," explains social worker Vivian Mirkinson, "they have taken a large step in acknowledging that their child is retarded and what it means in their lives." If the diagnosis of Down's syndrome has been made but no chromosome study has yet confirmed it, the test is performed at the Genetics Laboratory of the North Shore Hospital, Manhasset, New York. "This laboratory is not for research," says Dr. Arthur E. Mirkinson, physician in charge, "but for services to people in the community."

An evening spent with a segment of the community touched by Down's syndrome demonstrates how the clinic tries to achieve that goal. The setting is a group session to which mothers, fathers, sisters, brothers, and other interested relatives of the affected child are invited. The group meets in the evening or on Sunday morning, to permit those not free during the working day to attend. All present this evening have a common problem—a trisomy No. 21 child in the family. Dr. Mirkinson's explanation illustrated with slides is in clear, explicit terms and remarkably free of jargon. He discusses: How did it happen? Could it happen again? Is it necessary that it happen again?

This evening the parents are for the most part in their late twenties and early thirties, still in the childbearing age.

With one exception (an older couple) all are eager to absorb the facts on amniocentesis, to ponder its usefulness and place it into proper perspective in their lives when they decide to have another child.

The questions are varied and probing, and each one stimulates another. "Are there more children born with the disorder today?" Dr. Mirkinson reminds them that it might appear so because such children are more visible since families no longer hide them.

When a child with Down's syndrome is born to a mother under thirty-five and there is no translocation, the event, for want of a better name is called "accidental." For some yet undetermined reason the woman from twenty-one to thirty-five who has already had such a child is more likely to have another. By the time the evening is over the families have learned how amniocentesis can monitor future pregnancies.

"There seems to be a nondisjunction gene in some families," Dr. Mirkinson adds, "and there may be children with Down's syndrome born to sisters, cousins, et cetera." In these rare circumstances, prospective mothers in such a family can also benefit from genetic counseling.

The message has been successfully communicated to at least one family of a five-year-old boy enrolled in the program of the Brookville AHRC facility. His two older sisters both announced their engagements within a few weeks of each other. At a family conference that included both prospective grooms, they decided to make an appointment with the professional staff so that the brides-to-be and their grooms could learn first hand what genetic counseling would mean in their futures.

"What are the dangers for our children?" they ask. With no translocation in the family and no other Down's syndrome children, they are informed that the probability of a Down's syndrome child is extremely small. The young people left the conference with confidence, hope, and understanding. Indeed, they were so pleased with the service that a few days later a large box of homemade cookies arrived "just to say thanks."

During the past year, eighteen normal babies were born to high-risk parents after amniocentesis and tests in Dr. Mirkinson's laboratory reassured them of no chromosomal or other genetic abnormalities.

These are the people whose behavior and attitude will succeed in diminishing the population of Down's syndrome individuals in the years to come. It is not only the immediate families who benefit, for a significant number of Down's syndrome children survive their parents and may deteriorate as they age to a point where institutional care will be required.

The financial burden is then placed largely on society. Addressing the New York Academy of Sciences Symposium, Terrance E. Swanson, Indiana University, projected a cost of such care as $36 billion over a twenty-year period from 1969 to 1989. Moreover, he points out "no one can put a dollar value on anguish, broken families, destroyed careers . . . triggered . . . in some families."

To be sure, children like Steven and Debbie have brought much love and satisfaction to their families in their brief lives to date. Nevertheless, the words of one parent at a group session are echoed in the hearts of thousands of parents of Down's syndrome children: "There is not one among us who would not welcome a miracle that could change it all for us."

Until that miracle materializes, genetic counseling for the mother over thirty-five, the carrier of a translocation, and the mother who has already had an affected child can fill the gap with hope and assurance.

4

Sickle Cell Disease

When Jerry was ten, he overheard a conversation about himself not intended for his ears. "He will not live to fifteen," the doctor warned his mother. The doctor was mistaken, for today at twenty-seven Jerry is devoting full time to the task of telling other potential victims what it means to have inherited a blood disorder called sickle cell anemia (also called sickle cell disease).

Jerry is not alone in his goal of helping to remove what he describes as the "stigma of innocent ignorance" about a condition which affects 40,000 to 50,000 Americans, almost all, like Jerry, black. Two million more are carriers of the sickle cell trait, which is virtually harmless to the person who carries it but becomes a handicap when both parents are carriers and each transmit the trait to a child.

Although sickle cell disease has been a fact of life (and death) for more than 100 generations, it has only in the last few years become familiar to the general public. Indeed as recently as 1968,

69

a survey in Richmond, Virginia, revealed that only three in ten blacks had even heard of the disease. With its designation by the President as a "target" in his 1971 health message and the passage by Congress of the National Sickle Cell Anemia Control Act in 1972, it was catapulted into a position of prominence that promised for the first time to bring new hope to the thousands suffering from the disease and new insights to the millions whose lives it touches.

But perhaps the most significant development of the 1970's is that for the first time in its history, the promise of a specific treatment may be in sight.

What does it mean to suffer from sickle cell disease? Jerry looks younger than his twenty-seven years. "Many of us do," he explains. "Sickle cell disease slows down normal development." It should be emphasized right off that the development to which Jerry refers is physical. Unlike many other genetic diseases sickle cell disease has absolutely no effect on mental capacity or development. A child so afflicted can be as bright and progress as well as any other child, provided his illness does not deprive him of the education and experience that all children need.

Jerry's condition was diagnosed when he was less than a year old. Frequent fevers, sore throats, and a failure to thrive despite his mother's unflagging attention alerted the doctor. Jerry was lucky to have been identified so early—not many doctors in those days were looking for the disease. His early years were punctuated by fairly regular and frequent hospital admissions. When his anemia was really bad, there were transfusions for the infections, antibiotics, and, for the generalized pain, whatever pain-killer worked.

Despite the periodic interruptions, Jerry was graduated from grade school only one year later than the class with which he entered.

"I was only four feet tall when I started high school," Jerry recalls, "and no longer shielded by the presence of other handicapped children as I had been in grade school, I suddenly found myself surrounded by what seemed to be all giants and basketball types." One bright event at that time was the reassurance "You won't be a midget, Jerry," made by the doctor after a series of X rays of his wrist bones revealed that he had not yet reached his full growth. By the time he was graduated from high school he had grown almost a foot.

His adolescence was marked not only by the upheavals experienced by healthy teen-agers but by the burden of his illness. At social functions he was more of a spectator than a participant, but he compensated in the classroom, where he usually came up with the right answers. Are things very different now? "Not too much," he replies. "Sure they admire me for my persistence and courage, but there is always the feeling that I am different."

Jerry did so well at high school that he was awarded a scholarship to a business and secretarial college. Like most other victims of sickle cell disease, he is limited to jobs that do not require excessive physical effort and that will keep him off his feet as much as possible.

Hardest to take are the episodes that he soon came to know as a "crisis." The pains are excruciating—sometimes in the abdomen, other times in the joints. Often he can recognize when a crisis impends. For about an hour in advance he experiences a drowsiness and lethargy that warn of the trouble ahead. While every day of the crisis seems longer than twenty-four hours, when it passes, as Jerry knows it will, (lasting never less than three days, but never more than a week), he resumes his busy schedule.

"A crisis can be compared to a heart attack all over the body," says Dr. John F. Bertles, of Columbia University College of Physicians and Surgeons and director of hematology, St. Luke's Hospital, New York. It may be spontaneous, or it can be triggered by infections, fever, stresses both physical and emotional, and deprivation of oxygen. Repeated crises may ultimately affect the heart, kidney, bones, and brain.

71

While it is true, as Jerry's doctor predicted, that a significant number of victims die in the first decade of life, the long-held belief that sickle cell disease is exclusively a disease of childhood is wavering in the face of increasing evidence that many sufferers do indeed live to adulthood.

In a report to a National Foundation-March of Dimes sponsored Symposium on Sickle Cell Disease in 1971, Dr. Graham R. Serjeant talked of the increased life-span among his patients on the island of Jamaica. While the death rate among children is still very high, some 200 victims are alive and functioning well in their thirties, forties, and fifties. In some families individuals with the blood picture of sickle cell disease remained symptom-free at thirty and were identified only after a brother or a sister sought treatment for *their* symptoms.

A similar observation is reported in the April, 1973, *Journal of the American Medical Association* about twenty-one men and women ages eighteen to fifty-five at a clinic in Mississippi. All lead relatively normal lives, are actively employed, and have a history of mild, infrequent, or no pain crisis. Indeed, their experiences are so different from the classic textbook pictures of sickle cell disease in adults that the author uses a new name for this exceptional condition—MSD, mild sickle cell disease.

Even for sickle cell victims like Jerry who suffer from infancy on, painful crises and other troublesome aspects diminish with age. For Jerry it means that the almost monthly hospitalizations of his childhood now occur only every three to four months. Among Dr. Serjeant's patients there was not a single hospital admission for a crisis in anyone over forty.

Moreover, with the new look at sickle cell disease more and more doctors acknowledge that the toll it exacts depends not only on the severity of the disorder but also on the conditions under which the victim lives. Poor housing, poor sanitation, poor nutrition, and, most of all, poor medical care all add up to make a serious condition worse.

If the tens of thousands of victims of sickle cell disease are living with a "stigma of innocent ignorance," it can be safely said (with one in every tenth birth in a black family a sickle trait carrier) that the 2,000,000 carriers are subjected to a stigma and ignorance of far greater proportion. The fact is that sickle cell trait is an *inherited abnormality, not an inherited disease.*

In contrast with the disabling and sometimes crippling consequences of sickle cell disease, the life of the trait carrier is relatively unaffected. "In general," says Dr. Bertles, "if you have the trait, you will not get into trouble except in extreme circumstances, such as a large loss of blood due to an accident. You may notice occasional specks of blood in your urine. That alone is not a sign of kidney disease. If you are a woman, you may experience a greater than expected frequency of mild urinary infections during pregnancy. And if you need surgery, your doctor should know about the presence of the sickle trait. It will help him protect you when you receive anesthesia."

Dr. Bertles is often asked about sports and the sickle trait. Must the carrier, as Jerry did in high school, limit his participation in athletics to keeping score or acting as manager of the team? "Absolutely not," Dr. Bertles replies, "there is no reason why he cannot run, jump, compete, et cetera."

A Midwestern baseball team won the 1971 World Series a few years back with a black pitcher with the trait, and at least one black athlete, a Philadelphia medical student, found the sickle cell trait no hindrance when he ran the marathon in the Mexico City Olympics.

An August, 1973, report in the *Journal of the American Medical Association* tells of 569 black players in the NFL (National Football League) who agreed to be tested for their sickle cell status. Among these professional athletes in one of the most demanding of physical sports, 39 (almost 7 percent) are carriers of the trait.

It has been known for many years that the trait can cause problems to carriers at high altitudes. Back in the forties in the developing days of commercial aviation, a number of blacks unaware of their sickle trait status suffered painful but transient episodes on airplane trips (enlargement of the spleen, blood in the urine, abdominal pain). But such reactions are the exception rather than the rule. In fact, in Ghana, where the incidence of the trait is very high, pilots with the trait often fly at high altitudes in nonpressurized aircraft with no ill effects.

Sporadic reports appear in the medical literature often in the form of a brief anecdotal communication to the editor, describing complications in individuals with sickle cell trait. In addition to the now familiar and rare difficulty in flight, they have dealt with anesthesia, medications, and mountain climbing, For the most part, recovery is complete and prompt.

The soldiers who made headlines early in 1970 in newspapers across the nation were not so fortunate. They were the 4 among 4,000 black troops undergoing basic army training at a mountain post with an altitude of more than 4,060 feet, who died during a one-year period. In each instance the death was initially attributed to the sickle cell trait.

There was a stunned reaction, followed by an outcry that steps be taken to ensure that no such tragedy could ever recur. Within months of the publication of the report in the *New England Journal of Medicine,* thirty members of Congress and at least one state medical society proposed that sickle cell trait be declared a basis of draft deferment.

When, however, scientists and doctors active in the field scrutinized the data about the four, serious doubts arose about whether the deaths were actually caused by the sickle trait.

Most skeptical was the reaction of professionals well versed in sickle cell disease—both black and nonblack. Aware of the benign nature of the trait for most of its carriers, they viewed enactment of the proposed legislation as placing an unwarranted stigma on one in every ten black Americans, as well as closing the doors to those who wish to serve in the armed forces.

The Department of Defense responded by asking the National

Academy of Sciences-National Research Council to study the problem and come up with guidelines. Chairman of the committee was Dr. Robert F. Murray, Jr., chief of the Medical Genetics Unit at Howard University and one of the most articulate spokesmen in the black medical community.

After studying and evaluating the voluminous literature on sickle cell disease, the committee concluded in February, 1973, that "there was no scientific basis to implicate the sickle cell trait in the sudden death syndrome" of the soldiers on the mountain. They presented guidelines for the Defense Department for the future—that all recruits be screened for a variety of genetic disorders, including, in addition to sickle cell, other hemoglobin and red blood cell abnormalities. Some conditions such as sickle cell disease and sickle cell trait in combination with other specific abnormalities should be a basis for exclusion from the armed forces. The recommendation is that recruits with sickle cell trait not only can serve, but can do so with very few restrictions. Among these restrictions are serving as pilots or co-pilots or other tasks for which the "performance of the carrier is essential to the successful completion of the mission."

It is as necessary to dispel myths about sickle cell trait among civilians as in the armed forces. For years every airline has had rules about not hiring trait carriers for jobs in the cabin crew. "We can understand this caution in selecting a pilot or co-pilot," Dr. Rudolph Jackson, coordinator of the National Sickle Cell Program, N. I. H., concedes, "but why include stewardesses in that prohibition?" Repeated discussions with the airlines brought about a change of rule. By the spring of 1973 United Airlines (employing 6,700 stewardesses and 400 stewards) and Pan American Airlines agreed to reverse this policy. In the not too distant future, Dr. Jackson believes, all other domestic airlines will follow suit.

Another area in which the trait has worked an unjustifiable stigma and hardship is in buying insurance. All evidence available indicates that the life-span is not shortened by the sickle cell trait. The carrier is no greater a risk than the rest of the population. Nevertheless, there are instances where insurance companies either refuse coverage or grant it at an increased premium. One major company does not insure children with the trait because of the totally erroneous belief that the "trait can develop into the disease." Discussions are now going on with a number of insurance companies with the hope that they will reverse a policy so at odds with the facts.

The most unjustified as well as the most easily removed stigma of all may be the one imposed by the carrier of the trait himself. Without a clear understanding of the disorder he often suffers a distorted view of his present and an unwarranted anxiety about his future.

You may be wondering by now what is the culprit in sickle cell disease, why the trait is so widespread, why it is found in the United States mostly in blacks, and what determines who can inherit the disease, who can inherit the trait, and who can be born free of both.

To understand what happens in sickle cell disease, you must first look at hemoglobin—the protein that constitutes one-third of the contents of each of your red blood cells and is responsible for the delivery of oxygen to every tissue of your body.

The normal red blood cell containing normal hemoglobin starts its journey in the lungs, where its hemoglobin picks up oxygen from the air you breathe, travels through the arteries with its cargo, squeezes through the small blood vessels (capillaries) into the tissues, gives up its oxygen, and then back into the veins for a return trip to the lungs for fresh oxygen. The normal red cell will cover about 175 miles in the blood vessels during the 110 days of its life-span. When it is aged and worn out, it is removed from circulation and replaced by new young cells constantly being produced in the bone marrow.

The normal red cell is well designed for its functions—it has a good surface to allow exchange of gases, a cell membrane (itself a site of much chemical activity) that encases its contents, and an elasticity that allows it to move with ease from larger to smaller blood vessels. At least that is the sequence of events for normal red cells containing normal hemoglobin. When, however, the directions for making normal hemoglobin are changed, the course can become stormy.

Just such a mutation arose several thousand years ago—a mutation that was to result in directions for what is now called sickle hemoglobin. Differing from normal hemoglobin in a very minute way, it is just as capable of picking up oxygen in the lungs and carrying it to the tissues. It is only when it loses its oxygen that the trouble begins. Under conditions of low oxygen tension, the sickle hemoglobin comes out of solution, forms a gel of tiny micro crystals, and distorts the red cell. No longer the usual doughnut shape of the normal cell, it is instead elongated and may sometimes resemble a holly leaf, sometimes a sickle.

Up to a certain stage this process is reversible, and with new oxygen added the cell is desickled and goes back into service. When, however, the fragile sickled cell ruptures and is destroyed, symptoms appear. When masses of destroyed cells clog small blood vessels, the much-dreaded crisis occurs. And if the cell destruction proceeds at a faster rate than the bone marrow can supply new cells, anemia develops.

For the body to make hemoglobin, you inherit two sets of instructions—one from each parent. If, like Jerry, you have inherited from each of your parents the instructions for sickle hemoglobin, you will have as much as 90 percent of your hemoglobin in that form. Doctors call him an SS. With such an overwhelming proportion of S hemoglobin, sickling can occur in any part of the body where oxygen tension is low.

When, however, you inherit instructions from one parent for sickle and from the other for normal (called A hemoglobin), each of your red cells will then contain a mixture of sickle and normal hemoglobin usually about 35 to 46 percent of the former. You

77

now have enough normal hemoglobin to function normally except in the rare and extreme circumstances which Dr. Bertles describes. You are a carrier of the sickle cell trait, known to doctors as an AS. While sickling can be demonstrated in your blood in the laboratory (in vitro), that is not a true reflection of what is happening in your body (in vivo).

Benign as the trait is to the carrier, it assumes a much more serious dimension when the time comes to rear a family. With 1 in every 10 black Americans an AS, 1 in every 100 marriages can bring together 2 AS. (This also means that 99 of 100 marriages will be free of the danger.) In each pregnancy each AS parent can, purely by chance, transmit either the A gene or the S gene. If it is the A from each, the child will be AA and make only normal hemoglobin. If one parent transmits the A and the other the S, the child will then, like the parent, be an AS—a carrier of the trait. When, however, both parents transmit the S, the child with a double dose of the sickle gene will be an SS—a victim of sickle cell disease.

The risks with each pregnancy for two AS parents are one in four for an AA, two in four for an AS, and one in four for an SS.

When an AS marries an AA, *none* of the children can be an SS. There is, however, a 50 percent risk in each pregnancy that the child will be an AS. When an SS has children, none of the children can be AA. It depends on what the other parent is. If he or she is AA, all the children will be AS—carriers of the trait. Should an SS marry an AS, the risk for any one child inheriting SS is one in two with an equal chance of being an AS.

Various theories have been suggested for the origin of the sickle mutation. Some say it arose in southern India and was brought to eastern Africa in prehistoric migration. Others speculate that it started in the Arabian Peninsula and spread to Africa with early cattle herders. It is not known if it occurred independently in Europe, Asia, and Africa, but it is known that in Africa it appeared on the east coast first and spread to the west coast, the origin of most of America's black population.

If, as you know, a mutation happens only by chance and can take place any time in history and any place in the world, why has the sickle mutation persisted in some populations for millennia?

A map of the world and a look at those areas where the sickle cell is most prevalent provides the first clue. Those populations with a large incidence of sickling lived in areas where malaria was rampant—the west coast bulge of Africa, central equatorial Africa, parts of Greece, and southern India. About 1.75 billion people live in areas where malaria was widespread in the past. About 0.75 billion still lived where malaria is only partially controlled.

Was it possible that the sickle mutation conferred an increased protection against malaria? The circumstantial evidence suggested it. Clearly the SS child would succumb to the malaria as he does to other infections even more frequently than the AA child. (In Zambia today with a low standard of medical care, half of all children with sickle cell disease die before the age of three.) But, among those *surviving* malaria, an astonishing number had the sickle cell *trait,* as high as 20 to 40 percent in some regions.

In one study of a population where the incidence of sickle trait was known to be close to 25 percent, among 100 children who died of malaria, only *1* had the trait. In another study of children who died of cerebral malaria (malarial infection of the brain) not a single victim had the trait.

How the environment shapes the survival of the sickle cell trait at the same time that the trait helps survival of its possessor is illustrated in the West Indies. In the seventeenth century the Dutch brought many slaves from the African Gold Coast to their New World colonies. Some were sent to Surinam and others to Curaçao. When their descendants were studied three centuries later, it was found that the sickle trait was very much higher in Surinam than in Curaçao, despite the common ancestry with the same genetic endowment. The explanation? Surinam was a malarious region; Curaçao was not. And so in the former whoever

79

had the sickle trait had a better chance of surviving malaria and lived to transmit the trait to his offspring.

Despite the mass of circumstantial evidence, some scientists remained skeptical, for no one had come up with data to explain how an AS cell fought malaria. Does the AS individual develop a special kind of immunity? Does the malaria parasite shun the AS cell? Does the malaria parasite invade the AS cell as it does a normal cell and meet destruction there?

Attempts to answer these questions were fruitless until Professor Lucio Luzzatto and his colleagues at the University College Hospital, Ibadan, Nigeria, tackled the problem. In a report in *The Lancet* in February, 1970, they reported that the malaria parasite does indeed invade the AS cell. Once parasitized, the invaded cell sickles with much greater frequency than the intact red blood cell. The sickled cell, no longer useful to the body, is swiftly removed from the circulation and with it the entrapped malaria.

The sickle cell mutation, while it has meant death for thousands from sickle cell disease, has meant life for millions with sickle cell trait.

Doctors in Mediterranean Europe, southern Arabia, and India, as well as their counterparts in tribal Africa, must have been familiar with the symptoms, behavior, and fate of sickle cell victims for centuries, but it was not until the beginning of the twentiety century that a doctor in Midwestern America learned for the first time that a bizarre-looking red blood cell was the basis for it all.

In 1904 a West Indian black student in Chicago consulted the noted heart specialist Dr. James B. Herrick, seeking relief from a chronic illness that included, over a period of years, shortness of breath, heart palpitations, scars from recurrent ulcers in his legs, dark urine, sporadic pain in his abdomen and general weakness. In all his wide clinical experience Dr. Herrick had never seen a similar case. Nor could he find any description of it in the medical literature.

He was even more puzzled when he examined the young man's blood cells under the microscope. The red blood cells instead of the usual doughnut disk shape were odd-looking, resembling crescents or sickles. He did not know what caused the distortion or how the distortion caused the complex and life-threatening consequences.

At that time Dr. Herrick had no way of knowing that this condition was not unique to his patient, that it affected not only tens of thousands of blacks in America but was a significant cause of death of black children in parts of Africa. And, as time went by, it was learned that it affected nonblacks as well in some areas of Greece, Turkey, Italy, Arabia, and India.

Dr. Herrick observed his patient for six more years before he wrote about him in a medical journal. Slowly other doctors also began to recognize the disease, and in 1922 it received the name sickle cell anemia. (Many doctors now prefer to call it sickle cell disease because anemia is only one of its many manifestations.) And as more patients were discovered and their families studied, the concept emerged that sickle cell disease is a hereditary disorder.

Although many doctors by this time had seen sickled cells in the blood of both SS and AS individuals, the nagging question persisted: What biological or chemical events in the sickler caused his red blood cells to become warped and distorted? The urgency of the answer was more than academic. The hope was that once the cause was understood the way would be open to prevention or cure.

What makes a sickle cell different from a normal red blood cell was discovered by a scientist who, despite a towering reputation for original contributions to theoretical chemistry, had never been involved with sickle cell disease until he had an informal conversation with another scientist. In 1946 Dr. Linus Pauling, at that time a professor at the California Institute of Technology, was serving on a committee set up by President Franklin Roosevelt during World War II to deal with current medical problems.

Also serving on that committee was the noted Harvard hematologist (blood specialist) Dr. William B. Castle, who discussed with Dr. Pauling the enigma of the sickle cell. Dr. Pauling suspected that one specific component of the cell was at fault: hemoglobin.

His suspicion was correct. Using a procedure known as electrophoresis, he and his colleagues proved that the SS hemoglobin molecule is a different molecule from the normal. The SS victim has virtually only SS hemoglobin, the normal individual has only normal hemoglobin, and the AS has a mixture of each in his cells.

Dr. Pauling presented his discovery to the National Academy of Sciences in Washington, D. C., on April 1, 1949. The title "Sickle Cell Anemia, a Molecular Disease" signaled a new era in modern medicine, evidence for the first time that an aberration of a single molecule can have such a far-reaching effect.

That same year Professor James V. Neel, already famous for his work in another hereditary blood disease, thalassemia, published his studies on the hereditary pattern of sickle cell disease. After examining parents of almost 100 SS children, he found that in every instance both the mother and the father were carriers of the trait. Each had transmitted the defective trait.

Although Dr. Pauling and his group established that an abnormal hemoglobin was the culprit in SS disease, and even located which part of the complex molecule was faulty, they did not at that time identify the precise nature of the defect.

Hemoglobin is made up of two substances: heme, the chemical that gives blood its color, and globin, a protein. The heme of the SS, Dr. Pauling found, was no different from the heme of normal blood or AS for that matter. The defect, therefore, had to be in the globin.

Like all proteins, globin is made up of a very large number of amino acids—574 to be exact. It seemed a formidable task to pinpoint where in the 574 amino acids something went wrong.

Undaunted, the Cambridge University scientist Dr. Vernon Ingram (now at MIT) undertook the challenge. The 574 amino acids in the globin molecule are actually arranged in four chains, a pair of 141 each (alpha) and a pair of 146 each (beta). By meticulous and painstaking techniques, Dr. Ingram found, in 1956, a flaw in a *single* amino acid in each of the beta chains. In normal hemoglobin the No. 6 spot on the beta chain is glutamic acid. Dr. Ingram discovered that in the S hemoglobin another amino acid, valine, occupied that spot instead.

To produce each globin molecule, 574 amino acids must be assembled in the proper order. The instructions for that task are coded in the genes, and a mistake in the DNA means a mistake in every step to the finished product. When the genetic code was worked out in the 1960's, it was learned that the code word for glutamic acid, UAG, differed in only one respect from the code word for valine, UUG. This is the site for the sickle cell mutation. Once in the genes the faulty message continues to be passed down from one generation to the next. There was now firm confirmation of Dr. Pauling's statement in his historic paper in *Science*, November, 1949, that sickle cell disease is a "clear case of a change produced in a protein molecule by a . . . change in a single gene. . . ."

A whole new world of research on anemia and other hemoglobins suddenly opened up. By 1972 more than 140 hemoglobin abnormalities had been identified. Many are harmless and probably would never have been detected unless researchers were deliberately looking for them. Others when present with the S trait increase the danger of sickling, while still others diminish sickling.

Most significant was the discovery that different kinds of hemoglobin develop at different stages of life: the embryo, the fetal, and finally the adult (A) form. At birth the fetal form is still present and during the first year of life is steadily replaced by adult hemoglobin. Sometimes the fetal hemoglobin persists beyond infancy, and when this happens in an SS, it can actually provide protection against sickling.

What this discovery means to two brothers, both SS, is described by Dr. Serjeant in the *Journal of the American Medical Association*, March, 1972. The eye can be a particularly vulnerable organ in sickle cell disease but was not for Dr. Serjeant's young patients. The fifteen-year-old still had 15 percent fetal hemoglobin, while his brother at ten had 8 percent. Neither showed any evidence of eye changes so common to their fellow victims.

With fetal hemoglobin just as capable of carrying oxygen as adult hemoglobin, it could be a great advantage if scientists learned how to change nature's timetable for the SS and keep it functioning into his adulthood.*

So extensive has been the research in hemoglobin and sickling that probably more is known about it than any other major molecule in the body, but the cure has not yet been found although there is hope that one may be soon. In 1970, when the general public in the United States was just beginning to become aware of SS disease, Michigan pathologist Dr. Robert Nalbandian called a press conference to announce his success with a new therapy for sickle cell crisis—intravenous injection of urea.†
Newspapers, magazines, radio, and TV acclaimed the announcement with wide national coverage.

Despite the excitement aroused by Dr. Nalbandian's announcement, the performance of urea, in the experience of other scientists who tried to duplicate his work, did not fulfill its promise. Other scientists expressed reservations about the safety and wisdom of the massive doses of urea he used. Because urea forces fluids out of body tissues, Dr. Nalbandian's procedure causes a

---

* The presence of fetal hemoglobin in the first year of life explains why most SS babies do not suffer the full impact of the disease during this period.

† Urea is normally present in the body in small amounts and passed out in the urine as a waste product of metabolism.

Niagara-like outpouring with a critical loss of fluids and other chemicals (electrolytes) that must be constantly monitored and replenished.

By February, 1974, the National Heart and Lung Institute (NIH), which had been supporting clinical trials of urea at six institutions throughout the country,* concluded that the earlier publicized claims for urea had not been borne out.

But as so often happens, the new idea became a catalyst to spur fresh thinking. So it was with urea as a treatment for sickle cell disease.

It was at a cocktail party in 1971 that Dr. Anthony Cerami, an associate professor at Rockefeller University and head of its Laboratory of Experimental Hematology, found himself in a discussion of the new treatment for sickle cell disease. Together with other scientists present that evening, he speculated about how urea worked and why such enormous quantities of urea were required.

Suddenly Dr. Cerami's thoughts flashed back to his days as a graduate student at Rockefeller University. "Whenever you work with urea," his professor had cautioned, "you will always find a small amount of cyanate in equilibrium with it." Dr. Cerami was jolted. Was it possible that it was not the pounds of urea that accomplished desickling in Dr. Nalbandian's treatment but actually the small amount of cyanate?

The party over, Dr. Cerami lost no time in getting back to the laboratory to put his suspicions to a test. He obtained samples of SS blood, exposed them to cyanate, and found to his delight that it was possible to prevent sickling in the absence of oxygen. Moreover, even after the cyanate was removed, the cells remained desickled. This behavior was in contrast with urea, in which cells are again subject to sickling as soon as the urea is withdrawn. Not

---

* University of Tennessee, Emory University, Duke University, Meharry Medical College, Bowman-Gray School of Medicine, Travenol Laboratories.

only is the desickling irreversible with cyanate, but it can be accomplished with a small fraction of the quantity required with urea.

So far Dr. Cerami's work was only in the laboratory, with blood in test tubes. The real worth of his discovery would come only with tests in SS patients. Could a sickle crisis be reversed? More important, could a crisis be prevented by use of cyanate? Would the cyanate slow down or halt the anemia that often accompanies excessive red blood cell destruction?

He had first to prove to his satisfaction that cyanate is safe. (It had already been used in another context in the forties with no apparent ill effect.) Together with his colleagues at Rockefeller University, Drs. P. N. Gillete and J. M. Manning, and with an emergency grant from the National Foundation-March of Dimes, they initiated a series of studies with animals to establish cyanate's safety.

Two years of experiments with mice, rats, monkeys, and dogs have not yet revealed any ill effects. Indeed, the toxicity of cyanate was found to be roughly comparable to that of aspirin.

Reassured on its safety, the three doctors were not ready to test effects in man. The first set of experiments were with blood removed from volunteers with SS disease. The red blood cells were treated with cyanate and reinjected into the patient. The question was whether the benefit bestowed by the cyanate on the red blood cell in the test tube would carry over once it was back in circulation.

Repeated trials demonstrated that this would happen. The cyanate-treated cell has an increased life-span, the level of hemoglobin rises, fewer red cells are destroyed, and the danger of anemia is diminished.

The next step was to administer cyanate directly to patient volunteers.

By May, 1973, forty volunteers between the ages of seven and forty were receiving cyanate. None has had any ill effects.

Despite the demonstrated improvements noted in the patients' general well-being, Dr. Cerami and his colleagues are cautious in their enthusiasm especially in controlling crises. "A crisis is a very subjective event," Dr. Cerami points out, "and only the patient himself can define it." Under such circumstances it is difficult to draw a clear picture. For the purpose of the program, Dr. Cerami defines a crisis as twelve hours of pain severe enough to immobilize the victim.

Careful case histories established that the average number of crises among his volunteers was six each year. With a daily dose of cyanate by mouth the crises of those on high doses were down to two a year and those on low doses to four. "Not all crises are helped," Dr. Cerami warns, "but we do know that in all cases the percentage of sickle cells circulating in the bloodstream decreases."

If a study now in progress continues to confirm cyanate's safety in long-term treatment, large-scale clinical trials, conducted by the National Heart and Lung Institute, will begin in 1975.

Should cyanate fulfill its promise, Dr. Cerami foresees the day when an SS victim can with a daily dose live a life free of pain and danger in much the same way that a diabetic lives with insulin.

During the decades of research in the laboratory that have yielded volumes of knowledge about the basic abnormality associated with sickle cells, progress in identifying and educating its victims lagged considerably. To be sure, there were physicians, both black and nonblack, who were deeply involved, but for the most part its status in the professional and general community reflected ignorance and apathy. Some black leaders, including physicians, wanted to keep a "low profile" for fear of attaching a stigma to an already-stigmatized segment of the population. (They were not completely wrong, as evidenced by some of the events described earlier in the chapter.)

Among those who have consistently maintained a vigorous plea for more exposure and more attention to SS disease is Medical College of Virginia's Dr. Robert B. Scott. He contrasted the support given to SS disease with that given other genetic diseases of comparable frequency, such as cystic fibrosis and muscular dystrophy, or those far less prevalent, such as PKU. Sickle cell ranked lowest in research grants awarded by the government for the study of childhood diseases. "These data," says Dr. Scott, "argue for the need for support for sickle cell anemia and the need for increased priority by both the public and the health professions."

The support Dr. Scott sought became available from government funds with $6,000,000 in 1971 (up $5,000,000 over 1970), $9,000,000 in 1972, and $15,000,000 million in 1973. There was a sudden upsurge of activity: test every black, discover a sickler wherever he is, warn him, alert him, and, as far as possible, reassure him. It was a cause that could unify blacks who were wide apart on many other issues, such as the Urban League, NAACP, and Black Panthers.

In twenty-nine states legislation calling for mandatory screening of blacks was hastily drawn. California, Indiana, Massachusetts, New York, Illinois, Kentucky, Georgia, Virginia, and Louisiana enacted such laws. The City Council in Washington, D.C., found it necessary to label sickle cell disease "communicable" in order to pass the measure. Some states made no provision for counseling to accompany the screening.

Targets of the screening for the most part are children before they are permitted to enter school and young couples seeking a marriage license. Two states—Georgia and Kentucky—mandate SS screening for newborns.

Who should be screened, under what circumstances, and at what stage of life remains a controversial issue.

Yale University Professor of Pediatrics Dr. Howard A. Pearson is screening all black and Puerto Rican newborns for abnormal hemoglobin, including SS. He cites the three babies who died suddenly in their first year of life—the first inkling of SS disease, the severe infection and anemia that overwhelmed them. "SS disease is a serious illness, and identifying it at birth (in cord blood) is a valid medical goal," Dr. Pearson maintains. Knowing about it can alert the parent to seek prompt attention at the first hint of trouble. Dr. Pearson also emphasizes that his program does not include a follow-up on AS, since to carry the trait is *not a medical problem for a baby.*

Newborn children in New York State will also be screened for SS disease if proposed legislation for detection of seven genetic disorders becomes law.

The screening of school-age children to find mostly AS has come under widespread attack. Parents often do not understand the significance of the trait and tend to treat the children as if they are ill. Several follow-up studies reveal that in many families the confusion has generated unwarranted apprehension in the parents and unjustified restriction of activities of their AS children.

There is widespread consensus, however, that identification of the AS *is desirable* and *important* when the time comes to rear a family. Even then, a screening program is justified only if it is voluntary, confidential, accompanied by immediate and meaningful counseling, and clearly understood by those being screened and those doing the screening.

Claudia first heard about sickle cell disease in a freshman biology class when her instructor made a fleeting reference to it. She does not remember in what context it came up. Her next experience with it was an agitated call from her twin sister, married and the mother of a year-old son. "The baby is positive for sickle cell," Angela cried, "and they want you down for testing as soon as possible."

She was understandably dismayed—what did it mean to be positive for sickle cell? She had seen the baby only three days before, and he had been as usual playful, energetic, and robust. As for the urgency in her being tested, she recalled a vague connection between sickle and heredity. If the baby inherited his "positive" from his mother, she as the mother's identical twin would then be positive, too.

The baby had been tested on a mobile truck parked near the neighborhood playground, offering screening for lead poisoning and sickle cell disease. For their own tests Claudia and Angela went to the local hospital clinic that sponsored the program. Both were found to be AS—carriers of the trait. That was clear, but what was not clear even after the "counseling" session was what it means to be an AS. They were told that the baby had only the trait, but they would have to watch him for the next eight months before they were sure he was not an SS. (In fact, it is possible to find out immediately with an appropriate test.)

Almost a year was to elapse before they were informed that the baby was in no danger; he had only the trait. "I was nervous about myself too," Claudia admits. "If the baby's 'trait' could turn out to be sickle disease, maybe it could happen to me also."

Despite the less than perfect performance of the screening program, Claudia and Angela learned something about themselves that was to be of major importance in their future. When Claudia marries, she will want to know before planning a family if her husband is an AS too. Aware that such a combination carries a one in four risk of a baby with sickle cell disease, Claudia says, "We shall decide at that time whether to opt for the three in four chance of a normal baby (as some are doing today) or find some other solution. There might be a good treatment by then," she hopes. "As for changing our wedding plans because of it, I doubt it."

For Angela the decision had to be made *today*. When her husband was tested, they learned that George too is an AS. They were lucky with the first baby; only one of them had transmitted the defective gene. Are they willing to take the risk that the next baby might not be so lucky and inherit the defective gene from both of them? Much as they would like at least one more child of their own, they refuse to take the gamble.

"No more pregnancies" is their firm decision. They recognize how devastating a chronically ill child can be to a young family with limited resources and with hopes for a better future. And although they are not thinking of it at the moment, they know that when they are ready, adoption can provide the healthy child they want.

Genetic counseling with sickle cell disease is limited largely to what Angela and George have received: give them the facts; explain the risks; describe the considerable advances made in managing a child with SS disease. Ideally it should also include guidance in medical and educational services available to a chronically ill and often disabled child. The decision then is one for the parents alone to make.

Not yet available is a safe and effective procedure to identify an SS baby during pregnancy (as in Tay-Sachs disease) so that the pregnancy can be interrupted if such is the parents' decision. A report in the *New England Medical Journal,* July, 1972, by a Harvard research team describes their success in detecting the sickle gene in the fetus and suggests the potential for prenatal diagnosis. But to do so requires a blood sample from the fetus (unlike other prenatal testing that can be done with cells shed by the fetus into the amniotic fluid). Encouraging progress in accomplishing this safely is also reported and may not be far off.

Nevertheless, extensive research along these lines has a relatively low priority at the present time. While there are many AS couples, especially those who already have an SS child, who will eagerly accept the opportunity to monitor a pregnancy, there are probably others who would not.

Unlike Tay-Sachs disease, in which mental and physical deterioration, paralysis, and early death are inevitable, the SS child is mentally normal and, with proper care, has a chance to grow and function adequately. An increasing number of SS women are now successfully bearing babies with relatively little risk to themselves or their offspring, in contrast with the statistics in the past giving an SS mother less than an even chance to survive pregnancy and delivery.

91

No matter what the issues are that divide the experts, they all agree that the first step of a screening program must be education—both of those being screened and those doing the screening. (Indeed, it has been suggested by some that until this has been achieved, it might be wise to declare a moratorium.)

To accomplish this, the National Sickle Cell Disease Program has set up twenty-six centers for screening and education, which incidentally, also pick up other information about the participants' health—infections, failure to grow, malnutrition, etc. Designed as demonstration projects, some are in cities, others in rural areas; some administered by hospitals, medical schools, or health departments. A few, such as in Jackson, Mississippi, and the Eastern Shore of Maryland, are what one official calls "free-standing"—community-based. It is hoped their experiences will provide guidelines to the rest of the country.

Scientists have also defined a host of unanswered questions about the basic nature of the disease. Why are its victims so prone to infections? What is the whole story of the structure of the SS cell? What in the victim's blood contributes to the logjam of SS cells in a crisis? Do the ubiquitous hormonelike prostaglandins play a role in sickling? Is cyanate the best answer to desickling, or are there other agents just as good or possibly superior? To help find these answers, the national program is supporting fifteen centers engaged in basic and clinical research.

But perhaps the biggest bonus to the black population of America is that the spotlight focused on sickle cell disease also brings into prominence other health needs clamoring for attention. "Now is the time," pleads Dr. Clarice D. Reid, pediatrician and medical consultant to the national program, "to put sickle cell disease back into the mainstream of general health care." Pointing out that the sickle disorder is only one of many health needs to be met in the black community, she views the burgeoning interest in sickle cell as an opening wedge to deal with anemia, malnutrition, infection, and what is increasingly identified as the most pressing disorder of blacks—hypertension.

Indications are that this is a direction finding increasing acceptance by both hundreds of concerned professionals and millions in the affected community.

It may well mean that in the future, as in the past, a defective gene that has meant death to thousands will mean life for millions.

5

Rh—A Matter
of Incompatibility

Harry admits following in his father's footsteps in his choice of college and career, but choosing a wife who, like his mother is Rh negative is pure coincidence. "Rh today," Harry points out, "is not the same thing it was then."

For Harry's mother it meant the grim tragedy of losing three babies after Harry was born—one dead three days after delivery, followed by two stillbirths. For Harry's wife it means that a single harmless injection given to her in the hospital when their first child is born will allow them to rear a family free of the threat of Rh disease.

The story of Rh is unique in medical annals. In one generation the age-old killer of newborns has been identified; daring and dramatic new treatments have saved thousands of victims; a vaccine is now at hand which promises to eradicate the disease completely.

For many years doctors were baffled by a rare and mysterious affliction that killed some babies before birth, others within the first few days of life, and left many survivors mentally retarded, deaf, or victims of cerebral palsy. Erythroblastosis fetalis, or hemolytic anemia of the newborn, followed a strange but unmistakable pattern. If it happened once in a family, it was likely to happen again. Adding to the enigma was the observation that the firstborn was virtually never affected.

The mystery of erythroblastosis was dispelled in the early 1940's by two scientists, both trained by the undisputed master of blood studies, Dr. Karl Landsteiner, both highly respected for their own accomplishments, and both frequently called upon as consultants in knotty transfusion problems.

Dr. Philip Levine was working in a New Jersey hospital when he correctly pieced together the mechanism of erythroblastosis. Dr. Alexander Wiener, co-discoverer of the Rh factor, correctly worked out its role. Ironically, their landmark accomplishment became the basis for a lifelong rivalry between the two men, still smoldering today.

The concept of the cause of erythroblastosis was first suggested by a Chicago physician who had herself lost a baby to the disease in 1935. Out of Dr. Ruth Darrow's despair grew a determination to nail down the cause of her son's death. The hours not spent with her family and patients were dedicated to erythroblastosis. Despite some flaws and limitations in her theory (she failed to recognize that heredity was involved), she was remarkably prophetic. Ruth Darrow's paper attracted little attention when it was published. Dr. Levine was not aware of her thoughts or her work.

Rh disease is not a genetic disorder in the same sense as PKU, galactosemia, hemophilia, etc. There is no defective gene involved. The Rh factor is neither good nor bad. Indeed, when Rh was first discovered on the red blood cells of the rhesus monkey—the animal whose name it bears—it was regarded as a good research tool purely of academic interest. When, however, it was identified on the red blood cells of humans as well, it took on a new dimension. Among whites in most of the Western world about 85 percent are Rh positive; among U.S. blacks about 95 percent; and among American Indians, Chinese, and Japanese, almost 100 percent.

When the offspring of an Rh negative mother and an Rh positive father inherits the Rh factor from his father, his blood is now incompatible with his mother's. Throughout most of the pregnancy the incompatibility is of no consequence to either mother or child, but when during the last weeks of the pregnancy or during delivery some of the baby's red blood cells escape into the mother's circulation, she responds to the Rh factor as if it were a foreign invader (like a virus or bacteria). She then builds up antibodies capable of destroying the Rh positive red blood cells.

The Rh baby that triggers the first production of antibodies escapes the disease because very few fetal cells cross into the mother's circulation until just before delivery. By the time she builds up a high level of antibodies it is too late to harm him. He is out of the uterus and into the world.

However, in subsequent pregnancies the antibodies still present in the mother's blood are pumped back into the baby's circulation. If it is again an Rh positive baby, the antibodies coat the red cells, rendering them useless. They are rapidly destroyed and the consequent anemia is the first step in all the other signs and symptoms of Rh disease—the pigment that colors the baby's skin yellow (jaundice), the accelerated production of immature red blood cells (erythroblasts), and the heart failure that kills some babies in utero.

In the United States more than 250,000 Rh positive babies are born each year to Rh negative mothers. Of these about 5,000 are doomed to die in utero, and at least 20,000 born alive but afflicted with the disease.

With the new knowledge about Rh disease there was new hope for potential victims. Rh testing soon became a routine procedure in all pregnancies. An Rh positive mother will have no problem no matter what the father is. An Rh negative mother and an Rh negative father are also safe. But when Harry's Aunt Dorothy was tested, she learned that, like her older sister, she was Rh negative and her husband Rh positive. Like Harry, their first child, a girl, inherited her father's Rh. The doctor knew it was her second pregnancy he would have to watch.

By this time it was possible to test for antibodies in Dorothy's blood as the pregnancy progressed. A buildup could be a warning of increased danger to the fetus and perhaps an indication to induce early delivery. Repeated tests, however, helped assure them there was no cause for alarm. There was even a hope that their baby would be Rh negative. Not all offspring of Rh positive fathers are Rh positive. If the father is a heterozygote—one dominant gene for Rh positive and one recessive for Rh negative —there is a fifty-fifty chance that he will transmit either. When the baby inherits his father's Rh negative gene and his mother's Rh negative, he is himself Rh negative and cannot be harmed by the antibodies pumped into his circulation in utero.

Although she was reassured by the blood test, Dorothy nevertheless approached the delivery date with a mild anxiety.

Again it was an Rh positive baby. To their great joy he showed no evidence of Rh disease, but their elation was short-lived. Before the baby was a day old, he became listless, his skin yellowed, and by nightfall he was a very sick baby. A blood test revealed a very high level of bilirubin, a product of his red cells undergoing destruction.

It was not the first time that doctors had watched a seemingly healthy baby at birth suddenly become jaundiced and go downhill for no apparent reason. Now they not only understood it better, but were prepared to take vigorous action against it.

If the Rh baby's blood destruction is not too severe, the breakdown products (bilirubin) are removed into the mother's circulation while he is in the uterus. He appears normal at birth, as indeed he may be. After delivery his mother's anti-Rh antibodies are still in his bloodstream, and they can continue to attack his cells. He cannot handle it on his own. This is the time when brain damage and sometimes death can ensue. Dr. Wiener was the first to recognize in the middle 1940's that only removing the baby's damaged blood completely and replacing it with compatible Rh negative blood could save him. Exchange transfusions are now a routine procedure in every hospital in the country. Some babies need more than one exchange for full recovery. More than 90 percent of the Rh babies whose blood has been exchanged have been saved.

Among them were many babies for whom the doctor had induced early delivery on the basis of a buildup of antibodies in the mother's blood. On the other hand, the mother's blood was not always an accurate measure of the severity of the baby's illness, and by the time he was delivered it was too late. Only information from the baby would do. The first to elicit such information was British obstetrician Dr. Douglas Bevis, who in 1952 removed a small amount of the amniotic fluid in which the baby is suspended in the uterus. When the baby was suffering excessive blood destruction, he could measure it with chemical tests. The doctor now had a much better picture of his unborn patient. The procedure proved safe for mother and child and was widely adopted.

The value of amniocentesis would soon turn out to go far beyond Rh. It was not long before it was discovered that sex, biochemical, and chromosome abnormalities are also revealed in the amniotic fluid. In the next two decades amniocentesis was to become indispensable in genetic counseling for a host of hereditary disorders.

With another new weapon against Rh disease the death rate was again reduced, but amniocentesis by itself was of no value to the fetus that needed help before it could survive early delivery. It needed healthy compatible blood while still in utero.

In 1963 New Zealand obstetrician Dr. H. William Liley reported the first blood transfusion to an unborn baby. It was also the first direct treatment in history to a baby before birth. Dr. Liley's repeated successes were sufficiently impressive for him to be invited all over the world to demonstrate his technique and share his experiences. The intrauterine transfusion soon became an accepted treatment in the hands of specially trained and highly skilled doctors. It even worked for a pair of twins at Cornell University School of Medicine. The biggest successes with intrauterine transfusion were scored with babies not yet hopelessly affected, who could be tided over by transfusion until they could be safely delivered. The baby who had passed the point of no return was still doomed to die in utero.

Even before Dr. Liley's bold contribution, two teams of research workers, each unaware of the other's involvement, were already at work on the prevention of Rh disease. At Liverpool University it included young Dr. Ronald Finn, his chief, Professor Cyril Clarke, and others in the department. In New York it was Australian-born Dr. John G. Gorman, starting his career in the blood bank at Columbia University College of Physicians and Surgeons; Dr. Vincent Freda, an obstetrician at P and S and deeply concerned about Rh since he had first learned about it from Dr. Wiener in his student days; and Dr. William Pollack, an immunologist at the Ortho Research Foundation.

Both teams had the same goal: find a way to depress the mother's capacity to build antibodies against the baby's red blood cells. Using two different approaches, both teams arrived at the same goal at about the same time—an anti-Rh vaccine.

The basis for the vaccine was the discovery that an Rh negative individual will not build up anti-Rh antibodies against the antigen if he is given preformed passive antibodies at about the same time. Four years of testing the vaccine in hundreds of Rh negative males established its safety and efficacy.*

Now the Rh negative mother who has just had a baby will receive an injection of gamma globulin rich in anti-Rh antibodies within seventy-two hours after delivery. The vaccine prevents her from building up active antibodies against the baby's cells that might have leaked into her circulation. In a few months both the passive antibodies from the vaccine and the baby's cells will be cleared out of her system. Her next baby, if it is again Rh positive, will be safe.

Neither the Columbia nor the Liverpool group had set the date for their first clinical trial with Rh negative mothers-to-be, when an unexpected event set it for them. Dr. Gorman recalled the circumstances during a recent interview at the Columbia P and S blood bank where he now is the director.

Dr. Gorman's parents, both physicians in Australia, were following his progress with more than parental pride. John's younger brother, also a physician, and his wife were living in London. Katherine Gorman was expecting her first child in February. She was Rh negative, her husband Rh positive. Knowing that the first baby was in no danger, they were not too anxious about the Rh incompatibility.

The prospective grandfather was not as complacent. He knew that his son John's vaccine could work only if the Rh negative mother had not yet been sensitized. If Katherine's first baby were Rh positive, and if she were to respond with anti-Rh antibodies, her opportunity to benefit from the vaccine would be irrevocably lost. He felt strongly that there was no time to wait for the formal program to begin. Katherine should get it the moment she could use it.

---

* David Zimmerman's recent *Rh: The Intimate History of a Disease and Its Conquest* is an unusual behind-the-scenes picture not only of the scientific developments, but also of the scientists responsible for them.

Did his father have any doubts about its safety? "Not for one moment," John recalls. He had given his own boys gamma globulin to protect them against measles when they were children. Even if the new vaccine did not help, he was convinced it could not harm her. And since she would get it after delivery, there could be no risk for the baby either.

John Gorman found himself in a dilemma. He and Dr. Freda were the only physicians cleared to use their vaccine, and the approval was limited to the United States.

The date for Katherine's delivery was drawing closer; the baby was due in the middle of February. Finally his father's pleas prevailed. In the last week of January John took the vial to Kennedy Airport himself. His brother had been informed which flight to meet at London's Heathrow Airport. On the way to the airport Katherine's labor started. The baby and the vaccine arrived within hours of each other. The timing was in the best tradition of the cliff-hanger serials of silent movie days.

The baby was Rh positive. On January 31, 1964, Katherine Gorman was the first Rh negative mother to receive the vaccine. Would she have been sensitized without it? Doctors knew that Rh negative women were not always sensitized by their Rh positive babies, but they also knew that the larger the leakage of baby's cells into her circulation, the greater the risk of her responding with antibodies. Tests performed by the Liverpool scientists after delivery revealed that a large number of fetal cells had escaped into her blood during her long and difficult labor. Without intervention with the vaccine the odds were high that she would have indeed built up antibodies.

At Columbia P and S the first clinical tests got under way in April, 1964. A close collaboration sprang up with the Liverpool group, and in the next few years programs in the United States, Britain, Canada, Australia, and Germany confirmed their hopes—protection from the vaccine was superb. By 1968 it was licensed for general use.

To the Rh negative woman who has not been sensitized, the vaccine can promise almost total protection no matter how many Rh positive babies she carries. She will need it again after each Rh baby. Every Rh negative woman who has had an abortion or a tubal pregnancy also needs the vaccine. It cannot help the Rh negative woman who has already been sensitized either by an Rh positive baby or a mismatch in a blood transfusion.

This year more than 350,000 Rh negative women will receive the vaccine. If Harry's wife is among them, she will know that whatever incompatibility she may have with her husband in the future, Rh will play no role.

6

Pharmacogenetics—This Medication May Be Harmful to Your Health

Porphyria

When a prominent British physician learned a few years ago that his sister was a victim of a rare hereditary disorder associated with severe abdominal pain, progressive weakness, madness, and sometimes death, he immediately tested himself. He soon learned that he too was a potential victim. Then began a race with time to warn all his living relatives, many of whom he had never met and some of whose names and whereabouts were unknown to him.

The disease is porphyria—a genetic disorder that can remain quiescent and unnoticed for decades, indeed for a lifetime, and makes its presence known only when unmasked by a variety of drugs.

The discipline that covers such situations is pharmacogenetics—a concept in the medical vocabulary introduced in 1957 by Dr. Arno G. Motulsky, University of Washington, Seattle. It deals

105

with the way heredity affects one's response to certain drugs, including barbiturates, sulfonamides, steroids, aspirin, muscle relaxants, antimalarials, anticoagulants, and others. Beneficial or harmless to most individuals, these drugs can be life-threatening even in small doses to those with the defective gene.

Unlike other genetic disorders, pharmacogenetic problems occur in people who are otherwise normal. If they never encountered the substance that is their nemesis, they would never know of the gene's existence.

The doctor's sister was fifty-seven at the time of her first attack. It was also the first time in her life that she had taken a barbiturate. Had she continued in what her brother describes as the "family tradition that taking pills is a weakness," she might have been spared the subsequent suffering that was far more serious than the excruciating backache for which the barbiturate was prescribed. Her legs became so weak that she could barely walk, severe abdominal pain was now added to the backache, and her behavior was so uncontrolled and disoriented that within a week she was in a mental hospital.

At the beginning no one suspected that her problem was porphyria, a very rare condition. As a genetic disease it should have appeared somewhere in the family history. Moreover, it was hard to believe that such an inborn vulnerability would wait to manifest itself at the age of fifty-seven.

What brought it all together for the mystified doctors was the appearance of her urine. Instead of the normal straw color, it was the hue of a rich port wine.

Porphyrin—the pigment in the urine of the porphyria victim —is the substance that makes blood red and grass green. (In blood it combines with iron to form the heme portion of hemoglobin; in green plants it combines with magnesium enabling chlorophyll to trap the sun's energy.) Scientists regard it as one of the primeval building blocks of life. In fact, the discovery of porphyrin molecules in meteors from outer space leads to speculation that chemical conditions for life may be present in other parts of the universe.

Most of the porphyrin in the body is present in the hemoglobin of the red blood cells, with a very small amount excreted in the urine and bowel. An additional small amount is made by the liver in a complex process requiring a number of enzymes, each performing with precise timing and continuity designed to maintain the normal low level of porphyrin.

When the body is challenged by a foreign chemical or drug (including a barbiturate), the liver responds by stepping up its production of enzymes to help deal with the drug. In rare individuals, owing to a defective gene, a deficiency of one enzyme leads to an overproduction of another. The mechanism is very complex and still not completely understood, but the consequences are clear—more enzyme, more end product. In this instance the end product is porphyrin.

So much porphyrin is produced that it exceeds the quantity that would be released if every one of the billions of red blood cells were destroyed at once. The porphyrin piles up in the liver, enters the bloodstream, disrupts the muscle and nervous system (it was two years before the doctor's sister could walk unsupported), and is ultimately excreted, coloring the urine a deep rich red.

For the carrier of the defective gene even a small amount of the drug is enough to set this catastrophic chain of events in motion.

While it is not known exactly how the excess porphyrin produces paralysis and mental confusion, much is known about how the defective gene is inherited. In contrast with most other metabolic genetic disorders which require a double dose of the gene to cause disease and are therefore recessive, porphyria can be transmitted by a single gene—it is a dominant trait. Affecting both men and women, it can be inherited either from father or mother. Another unusual aspect is that it is one of the few disorders where *too much* rather than *too little* enzyme is involved.

"I have always been interested in preventive medicine," the

107

patient's brother explains. This time his concern with prevention has a special urgency. Were his sister's children affected? It turned out that her son bore no sign of the defect, but both her daughters had inherited the defective gene.

Having warned them about the danger they face with drugs, he next thought of other relatives. Determined to locate them wherever they were, he started with his father's side. Everyone tested normal. Now he would have to repeat the procedure with his mother's family. At the beginning the task of finding them appeared discouraging; he knew the names of only about fifty, but he was certain there were many more. A chance discovery of his maternal great-grandmother's "Birthday Book" was the key to eventually tracking down 200 descendants of his great-grandfather, who had died in 1862 after two marriages. One hundred and fifty-one descendants were still alive, many living abroad, some as far away as New Zealand.

To each he sent a letter informing them of his discovery, what it might mean in their lives, and what they could now do to protect themselves. All were very cooperative in providing family histories and specimens for testing.

Tests revealed that fifteen probably carried the defective gene. At least one death among the relatives not diagnosed at the time it occurred could well have been due to porphyria. Another relative told of a sixteen-year-old girl who suffered a temporary paralysis after taking a barbiturate tablet. Recovered and warned, she will, needless to say, never take one again.

The sleuth doctor wrote in August, 1972, that "there has been only one acute attack of porphyria in the family since."

The professor himself wears a bracelet around his wrist warning of his disorder so that should he ever be treated in an emergency he will never be given barbiturates or sulfa drugs.

In another example a Columbus, Ohio, woman, determined that others with the defective gene should not suffer the "harrowing ordeal" from which she had recently emerged, told a press conference in New York City in June, 1973, of her frightening experience. Like the English doctor's sister, Mrs. Kay Wagner Hughes was committed to a mental hospital after being unsuccessfully treated by a succession of baffled doctors. The barbiturates and tranquilizers prescribed there made her even sicker and suicidal.

Once the porphyria was diagnosed, the offending drugs removed, and an appropriate diet high in carbohydrates instituted, she made a full recovery. (Mrs. Hughes had been on a fad weight-reducing diet before her illness, and starvation can precipitate a porphyria attack.) At that point, on her own, she contacted the National Genetics Foundation in New York City asking for help for herself and her family. Only months before her plea, a San Francisco scientist, Dr. Urs Meyer, University of California School of Medicine, had reported in the *New England Journal of Medicine* a new test that could confirm the diagnosis on Mrs. Hughes and could also detect carriers of the defective gene.*

The foundation responded by offering to make the testing and genetic counseling available to all the relatives she could assemble. "I wish I could write to all of you that we had inherited a million dollars," she wrote to them, "but that is not what we have inherited. Half of us [may] have a hereditary disease called porphyria." She invited them to a pot-luck dinner with a free test as a "fringe benefit." Her invitation was accepted by fifty-two. Dr. Meyer flew to Ohio, arranged for the testing and counseling, and discovered fifteen members of the family who were to learn for the first time that they too bore the defective gene.

Dr. Meyer disclosed that a similar testing program would be made available to families of anyone found to have the disease. All that is required is for the family or the physician to contact the

---

* There are several forms of porphyria, each with distinct biochemical characteristics and each probably associated with a different defective gene. Dr. Meyer's new test is specific for AIP (acute intermittent porphyria), Mrs. Hughes' type.

National Genetics Foundation, whose services are available in a national network of forty-six centers.

While porphyria is a very rare disease in most of the world (about 1 in 100,000 in the United States), there is at least one area where 1 in 250 may be a potential victim. When Dr. Geoffrey Dean emigrated to South Africa from England in 1947, he encountered the problem for the first time in his career. After identifying his first patient with the disorder, he was confident he would probably never see another case again. No more than two weeks later however it happened again. This time a nineteen-year-old nurse had taken a barbiturate on her own. In the next eighteen months he saw eleven more patients—all with porphyria and all very ill.

At this time Dr. Dean embarked on what he describes as a "detective story that has taken me to many countries and back 300 years to the time of the first free burghers of the Dutch East Indies Company." The search took twenty-one years during which time he turned up at least 10,000 South Africans, descendants of a single Dutch couple who had met and married in South Africa (Cape of Good Hope) in 1688.

Apparently the defective gene was present right from the start but, with the exception of instances of skin sensitivity, caused no discernible damage. They were extremely prolific people; families of twelve or thirteen children were the rule. All seemed to have lived out their lives with no mishap attributable to the genetic defect. It was not until the turn of the century when sedative drugs like barbiturates and sulphonal became available that the gene manifested its sinister consequences.

Acute porphyria can also occur spontaneously and unrelated to a drug. Little is known about exactly what the trigger is, but scientists suspect that the body itself may produce it. Because episodes of porphyria are more frequent in women than in men, because they rarely occur before puberty and seem to be related to the menstrual cycle, it has been suggested that the female sex hormones may be implicated. If so, it raises a question for susceptible women on the oral contraceptive—the pill.

The *British Medical Journal,* September, 1972, warns them that "from a practical point of view . . . oral contraceptives should be avoided by women who have a blood relative with hepatic [liver] type of porphyria."

To the porphyria victim who asks, "How will I know if a drug not yet implicated will turn out to be as hazardous as barbiturates?" Rockefeller University researcher Dr. S. Granick devised an ingenious answer. Because it is known that a number of chemicals can induce porphyria in the liver, he turned to liver cells of chick embryos for his test material. After exposing the chick liver to the suspected drug or chemical, he found that those capable of triggering porphyria give off red fluorescence in ultraviolet light. Those that do not are safe. This test "should be required for all analgesics and sedatives," urges University of Minnesota's Dr. Cecil J. Watson in the *Journal of the American Medical Association.*

That the course of history could have been changed by porphyria was suggested in 1966 by Dr. Ida Macalpine and her son Richard Hunter. In an article in the *British Medical Journal* they attribute King George III's repeated bouts with madness to "acute intermittent porphyria." Later they expanded on the theme in a book *Porphyria—A Royal Malady* in which they claim that the British royal family may actually have been suffering from this disorder for 400 years back to the days of Mary, Queen of Scots, and included among its victims James I, as well as George III.

The book attracted immediate and widespread attention. It was the subject of front-page stories in the New York *Times* and other periodicals. Dr. Dean's response to Dr. Macalpine's hypothesis was immediate and negative. "How is it possible," he asked, "that in South Africa we are able to identify ten thousand living descendants all bearing the defective gene, while among Queen Mary's descendants no such situation exists?" (Dr. Macalpine cites two possible cases and points out that the unique position of a royal family and its relatives precludes the kind of testing that is taken for granted in more ordinary folk.)

Support for Dr. Dean comes from Dr. Watson and his colleague Dr. Z. J. Petryka of the University of Minnesota. "One may hope," they write, "that to make such studies (clinical, historical, chemical), the living members ... will set natural philosophy high above the distinction of lineage. It would be indeed heartening for historians as well as scientists if the present descendants were to volunteer for these studies."

And should it turn out there are some among them with porphyria, their very lives could depend on knowing it.

G6PD Deficiency

Relating porphyria to historical events makes for fascinating speculation, but there is at least one genetic defect whose role in history has a more secure place. In fact, it serves as a genetic marker to trace migration of peoples before and during Biblical times. Like porphyria, it subjects its victims to a handicap when exposed to a variety of drugs and other substances. Unlike porphyria, it is not rare.

Today more than 100,000,000 people, most of them male, suffer from an inherited deficiency of an enzyme called G6PD (glucose-6-phosphate dehydrogenase). It is widespread throughout the world, including Africa, southern Italy, Sardinia, Greece, New Guinea, the Philippines, and China. In the United States more than 10 percent of all black males suffer from the deficiency, but the highest incidence in any population in the world (58 percent) is among Kurdistan Jews now living in Israel.

For some with the deficiency it means that common drugs including sulfonamides, aspirin, antimalarials, vitamin K, etc. can trigger destruction of red blood cells and anemia. For others it may mean that eating the succulent and nutritious fava bean can be fatal.

In the sixth century B.C., the noted philosopher Pythagoras left his native Greece with a group of devoted followers and settled in southern Italy. It was a mystical cult concerned with mathematics, music, and astronomy. Their loyalty to their leader ensured complete compliance with the ground rules he established even when there seemed no logical explanation.

So it was with his taboo "Keep away from fava bean fields, don't eat the crop, do not inhale the pollen." Pythagoras himself did not know the rationale, but he must have been aware of the danger. Among his followers there were probably many with the deficiency, and he must have observed what happened when they ate the bean. Some years later, fleeing from an attack by pursuing Greeks, they came to a field of fava beans. It was their only route to escape, but faced with the choice of breaking the rules of the community or facing slaughter at the hands of the enemy, they chose the latter. All perished.

Today, thanks to the growth of pharmacogenetics in recent years, it is no longer necessary for the descendants of Pythagoras and others with the defect to make such agonizing decisions. Scientists can now identify who is susceptible, to what extent he is threatened, and how to avoid the consequences.

Were the problem still limited to fava beans it may well be that not too much more would be known about it in the twentieth century than in the first century. It assumed a new importance however in the 1920's and 1930's with the development of new drugs that produced symptoms not too different from favaism, not only in the same people susceptible to the bean but in other ethnic groups as well.

The first clue came from the antimalarial drug pamaquine. Within months after its introduction in 1926, hemolytic anemia was reported in several black soldiers. In the British army while soldiers from the British Isles did beautifully on the drug, a number of Indian troops did not fare so well. Scientists were slow, however, in recognizing heredity as a factor. In fact, a medical conference held in Punjab in 1944 suggested that the difference between the two groups on the same drug might be attributed to their marked differences in body weight.

With the introductions of the miracle sulfa drugs in the 1930's and their widespread use for infections ranging from boils to pneumonia to venereal disease, a new dimension to the problem was added. Again reports of hemolytic anemia mostly in Sardinians, Sicilians, Greeks, blacks, and Oriental Jews. During World War II with millions of troops of all nations stationed all over the world the use of these drugs soared, and so did the reactions.

The solution came about in 1956 as an outcome of investigation of a new and improved antimalarial, primaquine—related to the pamaquine of earlier days. When the drug was tested in volunteers, some reacted by developing hemolytic anemia. In every instance it was a black volunteer.

Intensive investigations in a number of laboratories followed and the pieces of the puzzle began to fall into place. The drugs hemolyze red blood cells because the cells are deficient in a crucial enzyme—G6PD. The defect is hereditary, passed down from generation to generation, hence more concentrated in families and ethnic groups. By 1958 it was learned that the gene controlling the production of the enzyme is on the X chromosome, so that while a woman with the defective gene will not suffer from the deficiency because her other X chromosome has a normal gene, the son to whom she transmits the infection has no protection. It has since been observed that the gene for color blindness, also on the X chromosome, is close to the gene for G6PD deficiency, and so both are likely to be inherited together.

The explanation of how the enzyme deficiency results in hemolytic anemia in the presence of certain drugs is found in the inner workings of the red blood cell. One of its important enzymes is G6PD—one of the fifteen enzymes required to break down

114

glucose, a prime source of energy for the cell. During this process intermediate products are normally formed that are essential in protecting the cell from destruction when threatened by drugs and other substances. Without sufficient G6PD the red cells become easy prey. And when enough cells are destroyed, the consequence is hemolytic anemia.

By strict definition the red cell circulating in the bloodstream is not a real cell—it has no nucleus. Without a nucleus it has no DNA to dictate directions for making new enzymes and other proteins during its life-span of 110 to 120 days. Whatever enzymes it has at its first appearance it must make do with. A diminished and irreplaceable supply of G6PD means a diminished resistance to drugs—whether it is the soldier with primaquine or the civilian with the fava bean.

Here the similarity ends. G6PD deficiency is not the same for every one of its victims. Scientists today believe that the mutation arose independently in Africa, the Mediterranean, and other parts of the world (only the Eskimos seem to have escaped it). One of the most significant new discoveries about it is that there are more than *eighty* variations. Some, perhaps as many as forty, are harmless, some of limited danger, and some potentially life-threatening.

If you are a black American, you may be among the 18 percent with a totally harmless insignificant variant (A+). Or you may be among the 10 percent of black males with the variant posing a moderate danger (A−). Even with this defect you will probably have between 10 and 25 percent normal enzyme activity.

Should you use a sulfa drug or primaquine, there will be no damage at first. As soon as signs of hemolysis appear, the drug will of course be stopped. At this time only your older red blood cells (more than fifty days old) run the risk of hemolysis. You still have a population of healthy young cells in your bloodstream. Soon additional young cells with their full quota of enzyme replace the older cells that have been destroyed. As long as the use of the drug is not resumed, the disorder is self-limiting, self-healing.

But to be a Greek, Sardinian, or Sephardic-Oriental Jew with the deficiency carries a much greater risk. The drug or plant is not so selective in the red cells it destroys; both young and old red blood cells are hit. You cannot replace them so quickly; the anemia is more severe, the sickness more disabling. Fava beans as a crop have come full circle. With its full dangers to a vulnerable population recognized, its cultivation is now vigorously discouraged in regions of the Mediterranean and Israel.

The key to control and prevention with this widespread disorder is as in other genetic disorders—education and awareness, not only for your doctor but for yourself as well. Before your doctor prescribes sulfa or other drugs that might cause hemolysis, transient as it might be, he will want to know of the presence of the defect. But in the use of nonprescription drugs like aspirin and other common pain-killers, the responsibility is *yours*.

"Children in families known to have G6PD deficiency," advises Dr. Sanford N. Cohen, New York University School of Medicine, "should be educated along with their parents concerning the hazards of exposure to these drugs."

With a relatively simple and accurate test available in an increasing number of laboratories, it is now possible for virtually every member of a high-risk group (certainly of a high-risk family) to learn whether or not he carries the defect. In some community screening programs for sickle cell disease, lead, etc., testing also includes G6PD deficiency.

When the Department of Defense requested the National Academy of Sciences in 1972 to come up with guidelines on sickle cell disease, it asked that G6PD deficiency be studied as well. The recommendations in February, 1973, were the use of a method that distinguishes between the mild and severe variants, and the exclusion of those with severe variants from duty in malarial zones since they were in danger of suffering most from antimalarial drugs. And in contrast with disorders like sickle cell or thalassemia with implications for transmitting the defect, the investigating committee believed that genetic counseling was not indicated as a routine practice.

Like sickle cell disease, G6PD deficiency is found widely in the malarial belt of the world, but there has been little clear-cut evidence of its protective power against malaria. Recent studies, however, in East Africa showed that children with the enzyme deficiency and women who are heterozygous (one normal gene, one defective gene) have fewer malarial parasites in their blood, suggesting that the presence of the deficiency creates an inhospitable climate for malaria.

If there is still doubt about the survival advantage by the defective gene, there is little doubt about the historic survival of the defect itself. The most complete picture of how it has persisted for thousands of years comes from the studies of Dr. Chaim Sheba, until his death, in 1971, director of Tel-Hashomer Hospital in Israel.

Combining science, anthropology, history, and the Bible, he suggested that the origin of the mutation now found in the Mediterranean, Near East, and various Jewish groups was the ancient seafaring Phoenicians and mercantile Judeans. The former brought it to Sicily, Sardinia, Crete, Cyprus, etc., where they established permanent port communities for their seamen. Because they did not intermarry with the natives, the frequency of the defective gene was retained and probably increased. It may well be that the bearers of the trait in those island communities today are direct descendants of the adventurous Phoenicians.

To trace the gene among the Jews, Dr. Sheba and his colleague Dr. Aryeh Szeinberg followed their migration from the Biblical events of the sixth century B.C. to present-day Israel. From the time they embraced monotheism more than 5,000 years ago, they drew apart from the people around them. Some of their isolation was of their own choice, some imposed upon them by a succession

117

of societies that regarded them as inferior. Through the years, exiled and dispersed to many lands, they maintained the integrity of their own communities and with it their defective genes—G6PD among them.

In 586 B.C. the Babylonians invaded Palestine, as well as other small countries in their path, and conquered large numbers of Jews and other peoples, taking them back as slaves to what is Iraq today. A group of exiles were allowed to migrate farther north to Kurdistan, where they continued to live isolated from surrounding peoples for more than 2,500 years. In 1948 they began to return to the newly established state of Israel. This is the population with 58 percent of its males deficient in G6PD today.

At the same time of the Babylonian Exile, about 1,000 families fled south to Yemen. There they intermarried into the population around them. By the time they returned to Israel after 1948 the incidence of the defect among them was diminished to a mere 5 percent.

Another major exile of Jews from Palestine took place A.D. 70 when the Romans sent thousands of Jewish men back to Rome as slaves. With none of their own women available, they eventually mated with the women of Europe. These were the ancestors of the Ashkenazi Jews, most of whom spent the later centuries in Germany, Poland, Russia, and more recently Britain and the United States. Among them the frequency of the gene was markedly diminished.

While Jews of Kurdistan, Yemen, Syria, Afghanistan, the Soviet Union, America and modern Israel all share the same spiritual heritage, their genetic makeup, uniform in Biblical times, now reflects their historic experiences after Exile. So that while among Kurdistan men almost 60 percent have the defect, among the Ashkenazi the incidence is an insignificant 0.4 percent.

For thousands of years there was little more than speculation and superstition about this disorder. With the proliferation of drugs in the last thirty years, the dangers have grown. Indications are that knowledge of how to avert the growing dangers is keeping pace.

For a discipline that did not have a name until 1959, pharmacogenetics has come of age quickly. The first book on the subject *Pharmacogenetics—Heredity and the Response to Drugs,* by Werner Kalow, MD, was published in 1962. By that time the triumphs of the new science were not limited to drugs that can harm or even kill. New data revealed that heredity can also dictate how much of a particular drug you need. So if you metabolize a drug too quickly, it may be eliminated before it has a chance to work. And if you metabolize it too slowly, it may accumulate to an undesirable level in your body.

Such was the dilemma with isoniazid, a drug that had been around for forty years before it was discovered in 1952 to be a powerful weapon against tuberculosis. Throughout the years since, it has continued to fulfill its early promise and is still the No. 1 drug of choice.

Not too long after its introduction scientists noted that while the drug worked for everyone to whom it was administered, the fate of the drug itself varied in different patients. Some metabolize isoniazid quickly (fast inactivators), while others metabolize it slowly (slow inactivators). Fortunately the antituberculosis action is so effective that even the fast inactivators benefit from its action. With the slow inactivators, however, there may be side effects that can be averted with appropriate medication when forewarned.

Frequency of slow inactivators shows a wide variation in different parts of the world and in different ethnic groups, ranging from a low of 5 percent among Canadian Eskimos to a high of 83 percent among Egyptians. Europeans and Americans of European stock are equally divided between slow and fast, as are American blacks. American Indians number among them 21 percent slow inactivators. The ethnic distribution was the first clue that heredity was involved.

It was necessary to look further, however, to nail down the hereditary component. Studies on families, sisters and brothers, and twins * soon confirmed the genetic basis. To make the enzyme responsible for inactivation, you inherit a gene from each parent. What they transmit to you determines how you will handle the drug in much the same manner that you inherit the genes that determine the color of your eyes.

Observations on genes and drugs continue to mount. In some families members with heart disease handle prescribed anticoagulants in such an exceptional manner that minimal benefit is derived. For other families it may mean the difference between life and death when a normally safe anesthetic is for them an agent that triggers extreme muscle rigidity with temperatures as high as 110 degrees. The scope of pharmacogenetics today, however, extends beyond the rare family with the rare response.

Adverse reactions to drugs have soared in every society and every segment of the population. Indeed, estimates from several medical centers indicate that one in every twenty hospital admissions results from a reaction to a commonly prescribed drug.

In the past "it was assumed," points out Dr. Elliot S. Vessel, Pennsylvania State University, "that all subjects would respond similarly to the therapeutic agent." Not so—is one lesson learned from pharmacogenetics. The differences are more common than hitherto suspected and often more subtle than a frank deficiency or frank excess of a particular enzyme (as in G6PD or porphyria).

In search of new clues a drug surveillance program was initiated in Boston's Lemuel Shattuck Hospital in 1966. In addition to the customary data on the patient's chart—vital statistics, diagnosis, treatment, past drug history, etc.—a specially trained nurse tests the patients under surveillance for a number of genetically determined traits. The genetic profile it is hoped will yield new information not only on the links between genes and drugs, but also on genes and specific diseases.

---

* In addition to isoniazid, identical twins handle other substances (including alcohol) identically. For a view of yourself intoxicated, let your twin imbibe while you observe.

Instances of the latter were already familiar. What seemed to be a biological oddity when it was first discovered in the early 1930's—the inherited ability to find a chemical called PTC (phenylthiocarbamide) either utterly tasteless or obnoxiously bitter—was later found to be related to certain types of thyroid disease. It has also been known for a long time that there is an unusual distribution of blood groups (your genes dictate which one of four you will be—A, B, AB, or O) in patients with cancer of the stomach, duodenal ulcers, rheumatic heart disease and in others.

The first dividend of the Boston program was in the disclosure that an unexpectedly low number of group O individuals were receiving anticoagulant therapy used primarily to treat patients with blood clots. Did this mean that if you are group O, you are less susceptible to blood clots and possibly safer from that particular risk if you are on the pill? The question was sufficiently intriguing to expand the study to research groups in Great Britain and Sweden. In all three countries the focus was on young women who developed blood clots: during pregnancy, while on oral contraceptives, or at other times. The results were identical in all three countries. A group O woman is indeed protected from blood clots not only during pregnancy but also when on the pill.

Since the surveillance began in 1966, more than 7,000 patients have entered the study and genetic profiles have been drawn for the majority of them.

There are few aspects of life where your biochemical individuality is more clearly expressed than in your response to drugs. Much of that individuality is coded in the genes that make you uniquely you. Bringing together genetics and pharmacology holds the promise that any drug prescribed can be tailored for you in both quantity and quality. Just as important is the role pharmacogenetics can play in prevention. More and more the warning can be issued in advance: THIS MEDICATION CAN BE HARMFUL TO YOUR HEALTH.

7

Hemophilia—Not Only in Royalty

Queen Victoria's eighth child, Leopold, was so sickly from the moment of his birth in 1853 that his baptism was delayed for three months. Much controversy arose about the cause of the infant prince's illness. It was public knowledge that the queen had been administered a recently discovered anesthetic, chloroform, to ease the pain of childbirth. Critics in the Church of England moralized that "painless childbirth is a defiance of Scripture," and the charge was that the prince's illness was in punishment of that defiance.

The fact is that Leopold was a victim of hemophilia, an inherited blood disorder that subjected him to a life of pain and suffering, prolonged internal bleeding, and crippling caused by severe damage to his joints from repeated hemorrhages.

Leopold remained sickly during his relatively brief life—lame and limping to the altar when he married at twenty-nine, and dead at thirty-one, leaving a young wife, a baby daughter, and an unborn son.

Eric is a young American, born 100 years after Leopold, with the same disease. While much progress had already been made in understanding hemophilia, the treatment was not significantly advanced beyond Victorian days. Much of Eric's childhood was spent on crutches, in braces, and in confinement dictated by his disability.

But before he reached adulthood a discovery by a young woman scientist at Stanford University launched a new treatment which was to free Eric from his crutches and braces and prevent crippling in young hemophiliacs who start it early in life.

Indeed, if a list were compiled of genetic diseases which can now be successfully managed, hemophilia would rank very high. The dilemma is no longer "What can we do?" but "How can we bring the advances of the past decade to those who need it early enough to do the most good?"

What does it mean to have hemophilia? Contrary to the widely held impression that when a hemophiliac cuts his finger or grazes his knee, blood will gush in an uncontrollable stream, the fact is that simple external cuts are not usually dangerous. The real hazard is from slow, persistent internal bleeding. Prolonged bleeding into the joints of knees, elbows, and ankles damages the bones and wastes the muscles. Hemophilia can mean a constant threat of death from bleeding into the brain, kidney, and other vital organs.

Until the recent past few children who were severely afflicted lived to adulthood without repeated hospitalization and serious physical and emotional crippling. It meant fear and danger in seeking dental care and extraordinary hazards even in minor surgery. It meant (and still does for many) growing up with excessive dependence on family. For others it has sometimes generated rebellion and hostility at the restraints imposed. And because hemophilia, like other chronic disabling hereditary disorders, is a family affair with a heavy financial and emotional burden, its impact reaches far beyond the victim.

Not only has therapeutic management of hemophilia come a

long way, but as Dr. Louis M. Aledort, of the Mount Sinai School of Medicine and medical director of the National Hemophilia Foundation, points out, the emergence of the team approach, which provides the integrated services of the pediatrician, hematologist, orthopedic surgeon, dentist, psychiatrist, and social worker for the multiple problems that the hemophiliac and his family still face, signals new hope for all.

Knowledge of both the nature of hemophilia and its mode of transmission was described as far back as the days of the Talmud. The laws of circumcision held that "if a woman lost two sons presumably from the effects of circumcision . . . her third son should not be circumcised. . . . Likewise if the sons of two sisters had died from the effects of circumcision, the sons of the other sisters should not be circumcised. . . ." They not only recognized the presence of an inborn bleeding disorder, but, with uncanny insight, also perceived that it was transmitted through the mother and possibly through other women in her family as well.

The observations in the Talmud were independently confirmed in the eleventh and twelfth century by other Jewish and Arab scholars and in 1803 were described for Western medicine by a young Philadelphia physician, Dr. John C. Otto. He recognized hemophilia as a distinct clinical entity with a characteristic hereditary pattern.

By the time of Prince Leopold's birth the disorder was no longer a rarity to the medical profession, but it had never before appeared in the royal family, so it was not surprising that the court physicians did not make the correct diagnosis. Nor did any one know at the time that this was not the first child to whom the queen had transmitted the defective gene. Her ten-year-old daughter Alice, was also a carrier and, like her mother, was unaware of it. Many years later and thousands of miles away, Alice's defect would surface to help change the course of history.

Two of Alice's daughters were, like their mother and their grandmother the queen, carriers. The younger of the two, Alix, married the soon-to-be Czar of Russia in 1894, adopted his religion, and changed her name to Alexandra. Their first four children were daughters, the fifth was the long-awaited male heir to the throne—a boy and a hemophiliac.

When traditional medicine failed to help him, the distraught mother began to seek help from other sources. She started with a French spiritualist from Lyons and ended with the Russian monk Rasputin, whose inordinate power in the imperial household was an added provocation to a long-suffering populace more than ready for a radical change. The climax came with the Revolution in 1917 and the assassination of Czar Nicholas, his wife, Alexandra, their daughters, and their ailing son.*

For well over a century it has been suspected that the hemophiliac lacked a substance in his blood present in normal blood. The first successful attempt to replace nature's "omission" took place in 1840, when a London physician gave a blood transfusion to a hemophilic boy who had continued to bleed after surgery to correct a squint in his eye. It worked; the bleeding stopped. The eager doctor was lucky indeed not to have run into the problem of blood incompatibility, for this was sixty years before the historic discovery of the four major blood groups and the awareness that some combinations can be so incompatible as to be lethal.

Even after that hazard was diminished many years later, transfusion of whole blood had other hazards, not the least of which was adding unnecessary volumes of fluid to a patient who needed only one ingredient. The pursuit of that ingredient localized it in the blood plasma—a step forward, to be sure, but still not a satisfactory answer. What was needed was a reliable supply of the missing substance separated from the rest of the blood.

Scientists identified the deficient substance in 1949, but as often happens (as in sickle cell disease among others) the new knowledge did not necessarily ensure immediate benefit to the

---

* In "Royal Hemophilia," *Scientific American*, August, 1965, Johns Hopkins Professor Victor A. McKusick has written a detailed and carefully researched account of Queen Victoria's legacy, among whose twenty-five male descendants there were eight hemophiliacs. The experiences of the Russian branch was the subject of Robert K. Massie's popular 1967 book *Nicholas and Alexandra*.

patient. The work did confirm, however, what scientists had long suspected: The clot that stops the bleeding when you cut or injure yourself is the end product of a very complex series of steps. At least eleven factors, each functioning in a well-orchestrated sequence, are required. Production of each of the eleven factors is controlled by a specific gene, and it is possible to inherit an abnormal gene for any of the eleven, disrupting the orderly sequence necessary to control bleeding.

In classical hemophilia the most common defect is in factor 8. About 80 percent of all hemophilic bleeders are in this category sometimes called Hemophilia A. Another 20 percent are deficient in factor 9, sometimes called Christmas disease or Hemophilia B.

Until very recently it was believed that hemophiliacs produce no factor 8 or factor 9, as the case may be, until it was found that some produce the required factor but for some still unexplained reason it does not function. Despite the initial skepticism by some scientists, subsequent work in a number of laboratories confirmed that the genetic defect is not in the failure to make factor 8 or 9 but rather in making a product that is different in a minor respect but different enough to prevent it from performing properly. If good health is to be maintained, it must be replaced.

A research team at the University of North Carolina made a significant advance when they discovered that the activity of the antihemophilic factor (AHF) was best maintained in fresh frozen plasma, which remained the mainstay of treatment for a number of years, although it was not an ideal corrective.

Then, in the early 1960's while working in her laboratory at Stanford University, Dr. Judith Pool observed that plasma allowed to thaw slowly did not entirely dissolve. Much to her delight, the undissolved precipitate was rich in factor 8. For the first time a practical usable concentrate of the life-giving substance was at hand.

The superiority of precipitate over fresh frozen plasma won it immediate acceptance. It now became possible to have high-potency concentrates that were not only more effective against

127

bleeding but also more predictable in content. A number of commercial companies now make a freeze-dried product that can be stored in an ordinary refrigerator, but its expense at the present time precludes widespread use.

It was now possible to treat a "bleed" (an internal bleeding episode) with a syringe and a needle. No longer was hospitalization necessary. "Sure, I've put off taking care of myself when I knew I shouldn't, but I could not miss a final exam," admits fifteen-year-old Len. Now a call to the doctor or clinic meant that the material would be thawed and ready to be injected by the time he arrived there.

The next step was to move the concentrate out of the doctor's office and into the victim's home. When Len needs a treatment now, he need go no farther than the deepfreeze in his kitchen.

With home treatment a success the next step was to try to keep ahead of a bleed by not waiting for it to happen, but by injecting AHF on a regular basis in a program of prophylaxis. By 1973 the move into the home and the prophylactic approach had been accomplished with a significant degree of success.

Home care by patients with chronic diseases is not new. Diabetics have long been injecting themselves with insulin. More recently programs of home care for patients with severe kidney disease and on dialysis has become an accepted fact of life. Nevertheless, hemophilia poses its own special problem. Treatment requires injection into a vein, and the patients who will benefit the most are very young children.

Among the earliest to report on a home care program (1970) were Drs. S. Frederick Rabinor and M. C. Telfer at the Michael Reese Hospital, Chicago. In their 1972 report in the *New England Journal of Medicine,* they reconfirmed that patients ranging in age from eight months to thirty-eight years benefited both physically and psychologically. In particular, fewer of them lost days from school and jobs. Home care was a particular boon to some of the older patients who admitted that, in the past, they had often allowed days to elapse before notifying their families of a bleed hoping no damage would ensue, although it often did.

How did they like the new regime? Some had early misgivings, but now all are happy with it. They experience less fear, less anger, and less anxiety. With it also comes a greater sense of self-reliance. As for the skill of the do-it-yourself intravenous injections, all the patients agreed that the home technique was as good as or better than the venipuncture by the usual physician in the emergency room. (Home care was administered by mothers, fathers, wives, and in some instances by the patients themselves.) In fact, a brother of a hemophiliac was of the opinion that all hemophiliacs over the age of twelve should be taught to inject themselves.

Similar success stories with prophylaxis come from Stanford University's Dr. Jack Lazerson, who is especially proud of one young patient who now accompanies his family on backpacking trips in the mountains. Enough replacement factor for the month goes along with the other supplies.

After one year on a home care program of prophylaxis instituted by Drs. Peter H. Levine and Anthony F. H. Bitten in the Boston area participants scored a 74 percent reduction in absenteeism from school and jobs, a 76 percent reduction in outpatient visits to hospitals, and a 45 percent decrease in health costs.

Eric is one of more than 2,700 hemophiliacs in the United States on home care today. It was instituted for him after a painful, intensive, and often discouraging program of rehabilitation had taken him out of the wheelchair and put him on his feet. The challenge was to keep him that way. His experiences since then are a testimonial to the success of the home care regimen. Now a student at a highly selective Eastern university a few hundred miles away from home and family, he keeps his replacement factor in a small refrigerator in the dormitory. His skill in injecting himself is such that when he senses a bleed during the night, he can "slip out of bed, prepare and administer the treat-

129

ment, and be back in bed without disturbing his sleeping room-
mate."

One summer he used his newfound liberty to drive across the
country by himself. With hemophiliacs traveling more than ever
before for both business and pleasure, they can find an added
security in a directory available from the foundation listing clinics and doctors in more than twenty-four states where they can get
appropriate help should they need it en route.

Recognizing home care of the hemophiliac as a "legitimate
mode of therapy," the Medical and Scientific Advisory Council of
the National Hemophilia Foundation issued a statement in late
1973 putting it into perspective for the patient, his family, and the
physician. (The foundation through its fifty-five nationwide
chapters provides services and counseling to thousands of hemophiliacs and their families and spearheads research and continuing education for concerned professionals.) The statement is incorporated into a booklet that features a practical guideline for
developing programs of home care by both hemophilia centers
and individual physicians, as well as an explanation to patients
and their families.

With the description of the benefits of the program is included
the admonition that "home therapy is not for everyone." Not
every patient or every mother, father, or wife is desirous or capable of handling intravenous injections. Moreover, there is a clear
reminder that home therapy is not a substitute for continued care
and surveillance by the medical team. But for the hemophiliac
like Eric home treatment is the route that allows him to "become
an active and enthusiastic ally in his medical management rather
than a passive recipient." It is more likely to bring a family closer
together and to be better prepared to confront some of the problems raised for them by a genetic defect in their midst.

An increasing number of severe hemophiliacs are living to
adulthood and marrying. Moreover, not all hemophiliacs are
affected with the same severity, nor do all, as the Talmud suggests, bleed dangerously at circumcision. It is known that hemo-

philiacs with mild or moderate deficiency of clotting factor can lead normal lives for years and are diagnosed only after surgery or a severe injury triggers uncontrollable bleeding. No matter what the severity of the defect, all are in danger of transmitting it to their children. Sisters of hemophiliacs need to know if they are carriers and what the risks are for their children. Clearly, genetic counseling for the whole family is crucial in planning for the future.

The genes for factor 8 and 9, like the genes for G6PD deficiency and color blindness, are on the X chromosome, and during fertilization, the mother can contribute either one of her X chromosomes and the father an X or a Y.

The son of a hemophilic father, inheriting his father's Y chromosome, is free of the disease. The chain is broken. So it was with Prince Leopold's son born shortly after his death. Each daughter of the hemophilic father, on the other hand, inheriting his X chromosome, also inherits the defect, but because she has a normal X chromosome from her mother, she does not suffer from hemophilia. She is a carrier. The woman who is a carrier can in each pregnancy contribute either of her X chromosomes. The legacy of the normal chromosome means that both sons and daughters will be normal. When, however, the defect is the legacy, a daughter * will be a carrier, a son a victim of the disease. So it was with Leopold's daughter, whose defective gene manifested itself in at least one of her three sons, who died of hemophilia at the age of twenty.

Until recently the best tests available for carriers were not more than 25 percent accurate. In 1972 veteran hemophilia expert Dr. Oscar D. Ratnoff, Case Western Reserve University, Cleveland, developed a new technique that promises a 95 percent chance of spotting carriers.

When a sister of a hemophiliac learns that she is not a carrier, it is welcome reassurance indeed. For the carrier however, or the

---

* Only four women hemophiliacs have been identified. A daughter of a mother who is a carrier and a father victim can herself be a victim.

hemophilic father himself, predicting the outcome of a pregnancy is still fraught with dilemmas. Amniocentesis can predict the sex of the fetus but cannot reveal whether the girl is a carrier or the boy a hemophiliac. However, just learning the sex early enough to interrupt the pregnancy has allowed parents at risk to make decisions appropriate for them. Thus, with a hemophilic father, only a boy baby who is certain to be free of the defect is allowed to come to term. When the mother is a known carrier because she has already borne a hemophilic son, or is the daughter of a hemophiliac, or has been found positive on testing, she can choose to interrupt the pregnancy if the fetus is a boy. However, if it is a girl and she carries it to term, the child could prove to be a carrier, and even more dismaying is the possibility that the interrupted boy fetus might be normal.

Not until a test is available for the fetus as it is in Tay-Sachs and other genetic disorders will the burden of such agonizing decisions be lightened.

Others at risk make the decision not to gamble at all. One young doctor, a hemophiliac, is now the father of two adopted children.

Would Czar Nicholas have heeded genetic counseling in 1894 if it had been offered to him and chosen a wife elsewhere? Alexandra had already lost an uncle and a brother from hemophilia and two of her nephews were afflicted. How much did he know when the match was made? The noted British geneticist J. B. S. Haldane commented: "Kings are carefully protected against disagreeable realities. . . ."—a not unfamiliar claim of individuals in high office today.

Complicating the genetic picture is that about 30 percent of hemophiliacs are born into families where the disease had not appeared in the past.

In some instances the defective gene may actually have been present in successive generations of mothers and daughters who fortunately have never transmitted it to a male offspring. Others are probably new mutations. It is not known what triggers a new mutation, but some scientists have associated it with the advanced age of the parent at the time of conception. Queen Victoria's father was fifty-two when he married her mother.

One of the tragedies of hemophilia today is the wide gap between what can be done for the severe hemophiliac and what is actually being done. Two essential ingredients are in short supply: antihemophilic factor and money. If every hemophiliac in the country today wanted to go on a prophylaxis program tomorrow, there would not be enough concentrate to go around. Moreover, if there were enough, the costs would be more than the average family could bear.

Until the day comes when factors 8 and 9 can be manufactured in the laboratory, the only source is from human blood plasma. The ironic fact is that in the 8,800,000 units of blood collected every year there are ample quantities of the antihemophilic factor, but much of the plasma is discarded before the factors are extracted. The technology required to reverse this waste is relatively simple.

The cost of keeping a hemophiliac healthy is high. Few families can afford the needed $10,000 to $22,000 a year. And while home care is considerably less expensive, it is realistic only for a minority. Most families are unable to pay these costs from their own resources, and the money raised by private contributions and drives is still short of what is needed.

It has become increasingly clear to all concerned that only state and federal agencies are in a position to take on the burden. By the middle of 1973, six states—Georgia, Maryland, New Jersey, Pennsylvania, Tennessee, and Virginia—had appropriated funds for care in hemophilia, and Massachusetts, Ohio, and Rhode Island had bills in the hopper.

Promise of action on a national level was incorporated in an announcement of a National Blood Policy in July, 1973. Addressing a Health, Education and Welfare Seminar for medical journalists in Washington, Dr. Henry E. Simmons, Deputy Assistant Secretary for Health, acknowledged the plight of the hemophiliac. The proposed national policy is designed to produce

133

the best possible yield of blood products needed for health and survival and to eliminate the financial barriers raised against their use.

Where ample supplies of the needed factor are at hand, hemophiliacs can successfully undergo surgical procedures that would have been undreamed of in the past. Even a tooth extraction posed enormous problems. Recently Dr. Stanley K. Brockman, Michael Reese Hospital, Chicago, reported the first open heart operation on a hemophiliac.

Heartening as the new developments are, scientists are by no means complacent. Much still remains to be revealed. Why do at least 10 percent of patients receiving repeated injections of AHF develop antibodies that inhibit AHF activity? How does the nonfunctioning factor 8 differ from the functioning molecule in the normal individual? Is it possible to activate the inactive component? How far off is the laboratory synthesis of AHF?

One sixteen-year-old put part of the problem in focus when he said, "Don't worry about the kids, Doc, but help the parents with their worries so they can treat us like we were normal."

But striking as the advances are, the best that can be offered today is a high-quality stopgap holding action that gives Eric and others like him what all the power and wealth of the royal household could not provide for Leopold—a chance for an acceptable, relatively pain-free life. There is a long way to go, however, before the sixteen-year-old's plea to be "normal" is truly realized.

134

8

Thalassemia—Cooley's Anemia

When Susan's grandparents migrated from Italy more than half a century ago, they brought with them a heritage meager in material things but rich in a quality of love and devotion that was to help sustain the family in the years ahead. They were not aware of it at the time, but they also brought a hereditary defect of minor importance to them as carriers, but life threatening to at least two of their grandchildren born decades later: Cooley's anemia, one of a group of blood disorders called thalassemia.

A thalassemic child born the year of Susan's birth (1950) had only a small chance of surviving to adolescence. Few doctors then would have predicted that twenty-four years later she would be holding down a demanding professional job in a laboratory, taking advanced college courses several nights a week, and enjoying an active social life with friends and family.

While it is true that victims of thalassemia still have markedly shortened life-spans and survive only with repeated blood

135

transfusions, the fact is that giant strides in the medical management has not only prolonged the life-span, but for many, like Susan, has made possible a meaningful and satisfying life. Even more spectacular are the discoveries about the basic underlying genetic defect that accounts for the chronic anemia, weakness, deformed facial contours, brittle bones, and short stature so often associated with thalassemia.

The condition was first recognized as a clinical entity in 1925 by a Detroit physician, Dr. Thomas B. Cooley, whose name the most common type still bears. Within the next few years many more cases were reported both in the United States and Europe. Most of the victims identified at that time were of Mediterranean ancestry (Italian and Greek), and by 1936 a new name—thalassemia, from the Greek word for sea—was adopted. It has since been found in diverse ethnic groups almost all over the world.

The first suggestion that it had a hereditary nature came in 1938 following observations that the parents of children with Cooley's anemia, while not sick themselves, showed an abnormality of their red blood cells. By 1944 the genetic aspects of the disorder were firmly established. As in Tay-Sachs and sickle cell disease, both parents are carriers of the trait (thalassemia minor) and, as in other recessive genetic disorders, are probably unaware of it. When, however, each transmits the trait, the baby, with a double dose of the defect, is a victim of thalassemia major.

A seemingly healthy baby at birth, Susan began to show signs of the anemia before her first birthday. Her continued pallor, failure to gain weight, an enlarged spleen engorged with broken-down red blood cells—all added up to the suspicion of thalassemia. There was no history of any one else in the family's having been affected, but with her Italian ancestry the diagnosis had to be considered.

Laboratory tests soon revealed typical characteristics of the disorder—smaller than normal red blood cells deficient in hemoglobin and incapable of supplying the body with the oxygen it needs. Many cells had the familiar "target" cell appearance. There was then no cure, no medication. The best that doctors could promise was a brief painful life maintained for a few years with blood transfusions.

The dismal prognosis for Susan was only part of the shock for the young parents. The news that her illness was hereditary, that each of them had transmitted a defective gene, and that it could happen again took on a special urgency. Another baby was on the way, conceived before the thalassemia diagnosis had been made. They were now aware of the one in four risk of its happening again.

This time it was a boy—and, to their delight, free of the disease.

Their third child was born when Susan was seven. Paul was not as lucky as his older brother. Like Susan, he is a victim of thalassemia and, like Susan, functions well today. He loves sports and often joins his friends in a game of football. Paul has some well-defined plans for a career—someday he would like to be a doctor.

How realistic are dreams for a future for Susan and Paul and thousands like them? Much depends on how quickly science comes up with answers to questions that could not even have been asked in the not too distant past.

For the thalassemic today, the most pressing questions are how to turn the clock back on early death and how to enjoy life without being cast in the role of a hopeless invalid.

Scientists have known since the days of Dr. Cooley that the thalassemic red blood cell is severely deficient in hemoglobin and that it is also easy prey to destruction in the bloodstream. In simpler and more commonplace anemias the body steps up the activity of the bone marrow and releases new cells into the blood to replace those lost. In thalassemia, no matter how much work the bone marrow does, it can't win. The new red blood cells are as short-lived as the old, and the rate at which they are released never surpasses the rate at which they are destroyed. Indeed, so much excess bone marrow develops in the effort to produce new cells that it can no longer be comfortably contained and, as a result, deforms the bone itself. This accounts for the mongoloid appearance that so many thalassemics have and for the fragility of their bones.

Their hearts work overtime in just as futile an effort to pump more blood to their oxygen-starved tissues and become enlarged and damaged in the process, so that death from heart failure is a constant threat.

Unable to fight his anemia with his own resources, the thalassemic is then totally dependent on transfused blood. Today, as in the past, transfusions are the only therapy that works. The improvement is in the blood product itself: fresh frozen packed red blood cells, and in the new concept of how much and how often to administer it.

The traditional practice was to transfuse just often enough to ensure survival—not always synonomous with well-being. Growth lagged; energy ebbed. But doctors knew that more blood and more transfusions had built-in dangers of their own. Even without transfusions vital organs (heart, liver, pancreas, etc.) suffer from iron deposits released from broken-down red blood cells. How would the additional iron burden from transfused blood cells be tolerated?

On the other hand, what would happen to a child if the severe anemia were never allowed to gain a foothold? Would maintaining a normal hemoglobin from infancy on with periodic frequent transfusions divert the disastrous course of thalassemia and produce a normal-looking, normally functioning child?

Mindful of the possible disadvantages of such a regimen but hopeful that the benefits would outweigh the risks, Dr. Irving Wolman, University of Pennsylvania, started just such a program at the Children's Hospital, Philadelphia. In his preliminary report to the First Conference on Cooley's Anemia in 1963, he described some of the children under treatment. They were growing up with more normal facial structure, had suffered no fractures, and were in all-around better health. Greatest beneficiaries were those who were very young when HTR (hyper transfusion regimen) was instituted. Dr. Wolman emphasized that it was still too early to predict long-term effects.

It did not take long for other thalassemia specialists to adopt HTR. By 1973 similar experiences by others were reported to the Third Conference on Cooley's Anemia. Among them was Dr. Thomas E. Necheles of Boston's New England Medical Center, who observed after an eight-year follow-up "marked improvement in general health and level of activity particularly in those children who were . . . started when less than ten years of age. The oldest works full time; the others are full time students who miss no more than the normal amount of school, and two of the younger children are on athletic teams—skiing and tennis."

A problem as yet unsolved is the increased quantity of iron introduced with the stepped-up transfusion and longer life-span. No safe and effective means is yet available for its removal, although there is evidence that patients on HTR and not chronically anemic can deal with some of the iron on their own. Development of a good chemical agent to reduce the iron remains one of the high-priority targets of today's research. Ironically a 1973 plan to improve nutrition for millions of Americans by adding iron to bread is a new threat to any individual with the thalassemia gene.

Susan and Paul are both on HTR, and their continued progress reflects not only their medical treatment, but the ambiance of a loving, understanding family in which they receive no special privileges and no special restrictions. "Susan may come home from a transfusion," her father relates, "and if it is her turn to do the dinner dishes, she does them."

Each member of the family also understands what it may mean to him if he is a carrier of the trait. Often a thalassemia minor has a mild anemia throughout his lifetime and may be mistakenly treated for it. The fact is that he can function perfectly normally and live out his full life-span. Should he, however, be given iron to raise his blood hemoglobin level, not only will it not help, but it may be harmful.

The major concern, when both parents are carriers of the thalassemia gene, is the one in four risk in each pregnancy that the baby may have thalassemia major.

More than twenty years ago, not long after the nature of Susan's illness was confirmed, her father gathered together his close relatives at a cousins' club function and explained that they and their spouses might also be carriers of the trait. Their reaction was almost a unanimous "no—it can't happen to us." They have been lucky. All have since reared families; none has had thalassemic children.

Some of those children are grown and planning their own marriages. Recognizing their membership in a high-risk group, at least two prospective bridegrooms plan to be tested along with their brides-to-be. "No matter what the outcome of the tests," they comment, "the marriage plans stand."

While there are tests for carriers that are practical for individuals in a high-risk family such as Susan and Paul's cousins, there has not been until recently a simple, accurate and inexpensive test to screen large numbers of people in a high-risk population.

At the Yale University School of Medicine, Dr. Peter Mc-Phedran observed that when he examined red blood cells with an electronic cell counter, 25 percent of the patients whose cells were smaller than normal turned out to be carriers of the thalassemia trait (a fact subsequently verified by more cumbersome and time-consuming procedures). Because the electronic counter gives a printout of a blood specimen in less than a minute, it was suggested that it might be suitable for the long-hoped-for simple and inexpensive test. Dr. Howard A. Pearson, a professor of pediatrics at Yale and known for his work in genetic blood disorders (he was the recent recipient of a Martin Luther King award for sickle cell disease), gave the test its first trial in a mass screening program in a high-risk population.

140

The screening, accompanied by appropriate education and counseling, was offered on a voluntary basis to members of the congregations of two Greek Orthodox churches, 170 teen-age high school students of Italian ancestry, members of families where thalassemia had already been identified, and all Greeks and Italians who wanted to be tested.

More than 600 responded. Those whose screening tests raised suspicions received more precise tests. About 5 percent of the Greek population were found to be carriers of the thalassemia trait. (A recent study among Greek Cypriotes in London uncovered 14 percent carriers.) The frequency among Italian-Americans was lower—2.4 percent.

A significant number of the newly identified carriers of the trait can now be spared treatment for an "anemia" that needs no treatment. When forty-five were asked, "Have you ever been diagnosed as anemic and, if so, what was done about it?" more than half replied that they had in fact been so diagnosed. Twenty-three had received iron therapy for a long time, some by injection. Others were given vitamin B_{12} shots unnecessarily. One even received a blood transfusion.

The parents of two healthy children learned for the first time that each is a carrier of the thalassemia trait and that they might not be so lucky with a third child. What they received was a "before-the-fact counseling." For many in such a position the decision may well be no more pregnancies.

Not too far off is a test that will make possible the identification of a thalassemia baby early in pregnancy. As in Tay-Sachs and Down's syndrome, it will then be the parents' choice whether to interrupt the pregnancy, with the hope that the next will be a baby free of the disease.

The test for prenatal diagnosis is only one application of the discoveries about the basic genetic defect in thalassemia that will ultimately lead to its control and prevention.

Linus Pauling's historic announcement in 1949 of the abnormal hemoglobin in sickle cell disease spurred the search for comparable discoveries about other anemias, including thalassemia. Hemoglobin is a protein made up of four chains of amino acids—two alpha and two beta—each assembled from instructions coded in your genes. In the sickle cell a single amino acid is incorrectly assembled into the beta chain, resulting in a flawed hemoglobin molecule.

In thalassemia, on the other hand, all the chains appear to be normal in structure, but instead of a balanced amount of alpha and beta chains, there is a deficit of the latter and a marked excess of the former. Indeed, the imbalance is so great that many of the alphas with no betas to which they can attach precipitate out into the red cells, weakening them and hastening their destruction. It has recently been learned that the messenger RNA responsible for beta chain synthesis in thalassemia is normal in structure but for some still unexplained reason functions at a reduced rate.

While the most common form of thalassemia is a shortage of beta chain (as in Cooley's anemia), it is now known that thalassemia can also be caused by a shortage of alpha chains—alpha thalassemia. In fact, in one variation all four chains are beta with no alpha chains at all. What was for many years, since the days of Dr. Cooley, considered a single disorder now emerges as possibly twenty variants—each with its own constellation of symptoms and behavior.

The new look at the nature of thalassemia was accompanied by a new look at its victims and where they are. It is now clear that the disorder is by no means limited to Italians and Greeks and their descendants.

The recollection is still vivid of the excitement generated in the laboratory of an army hospital back in 1943 when a Chinese soldier, born in China with Chinese ancestors, was diagnosed as a Cooley's anemia by Dr. I. J. Greenblatt, director of the laboratory service at Camp Stoneman. Hard to believe was its appearance in a Chinese, and even more puzzling was the then-unknown phenomenon of a victim of twenty-nine in good enough health to be in the army. (The report was published in the *Annals of Internal Medicine,* February, 1946.) It was a portent of many such exceptions in the years ahead.

In the city of Jerusalem, thalassemia has brought together Jews and Arabs in a joint venture that could be a model for cooperation for the future on other levels. Dr. Eliezer Rachmilewitz directs a program at Hadassah Medical Center where more than 30 children and young adults—Arabs and Jews—are treated for thalassemia. He estimates that as many as 4,000 residents of Jerusalem may be carriers of the trait. A committee is now at work with the goal of educating those at risk about the meaning of the disease and the value of screening for carriers. Dr. Rachmilewitz tells of one Arab family in the upper Galilee where 44 members screened were found to have the trait and warned.

Beta thalassemia is also found in several forms in black Americans. For some it is a serious illness identical with Cooley's anemia. For others it runs a milder course often requiring no transfusions. About 2 to 3 percent inherit a sickle gene from one parent and a thalassemia gene from the other. Their illness is usually not as serious as a double dose of the sickle gene or a double dose of the thalassemic gene. Genetic counseling for them includes the possible risks of transmitting each of the defective genes.

By now thalassemia has been found in the Sudan, New Guinea, India, Pakistan, Nepal, Burma, Indonesia, and China. One of the highest concentrations of the thalassemia trait is in Thailand, where it is estimated that more than 350,000 carry the defective gene.

Dr. Cooley would not be surprised at the ubiquitous distribution, for as early as 1932 he wrote that "we are not inclined . . . to lay great stress on the limitations of this or any other similar disease to a particular race."

Where and when did thalassemia originate, and why has it survived among so many in such far-flung places? One theory implicates the Greeks of 3,000 years ago when their empire stretched from Sicily and southern Italy east to Asia Minor. Another theory has its origin in Asia Minor and spread again by the Greeks in their expansion westward.

Because thalassemia leaves telltale signs in the skull and other bones of its victims, it has left a record locked into the fossils of the distant past. The earliest such find was a skeleton from an excavation in Messina, Sicily, dating back 35,000 to 40,000 years ago. Other archaeological digs yielded evidence of thalassemia in two infant skulls of ancient Egypt 2,000 B.C., pre-Columbian Indians of ancient Peru, the Mayas of Yucatán, Indian infants from New Mexico, and the mound builders of eastern Arkansas. A dig in France uncovered a specimen dating back to Roman occupation. These discoveries suggest that the global distribution of thalassemia cannot necessarily be attributed to modern migration alone.

To Dr. Edward C. Zaino, the director of Laboratories, Mercy Hospital, Rockville Centre, New York, these clues added up to a hypothesis he presented to the First Conference on Cooley's Anemia, published in the *Annals of the New York Academy of Sciences* in 1964 under the title of "Paleontologic Thalassemia." Because the greatest concentration of thalassemia today is in Italy and Greece, he pinpoints the origin in that region. He speculates that the defective gene in the Messina victim had already migrated many thousands of years earlier from its origin in a valley in southern Italy on the shores of two freshwater lakes. The lowlands could have been malaria-infested, and if, as Dr. Zaino and many other scientists believe, the thalassemia trait protects against malaria (as sickle trait does), its frequency would have been high. Two land bridges at that time between Europe and Africa permitted migration and, with it, spread of the defective trait.

In a later era, when the glaciers to the north melted and the ocean level rose, the valley was inundated and the Mediterranean was born. Survivors in the lowlands sought safety elsewhere. Some migrated north to higher ground in Italy and Greece, south to parts of Africa, east to the Middle East and farther into India.

144

". . . in migrating into the near east and India, [they] could have taken their thalassemia with them," says Dr. Zaino. "The gene could have continued up the Pacific coasts into China, then across the Bering Strait into North and South America."

Since the last migration of American Indians from Asia was 15,000 to 20,000 years ago, their Asian ancestors must have had thalassemia before then. The thalassemic fossils in Peru, it was noted, were found only in coastal areas, another clue that the defective gene may have played a role in survival against malaria.

Dr. Zaino's provocative look into the past is only one facet of the unflagging interest sustained by those concerned with this worldwide disorder.

The fight against thalassemia was given a substantial boost in 1972 with the passage by Congress of the National Cooley's Anemia Control Act with more than $11,000,000 requested for education and research in the next three years. Probably no more than a small percentage of Americans were familiar with the disease when they read about it at the time, but to the dedicated and involved members of the Cooley's Anemia Blood and Research Foundation for Children, the new legislation meant winning a battle in a war whose end was not yet in sight. One of the initial goals of the foundation, started in 1954 by a handful of parents of thalassemic children. was to keep open the lifeline of blood essential to their children's survival.

Today there are thirteen chapters across the country, and while making blood available to every thalassemic child who needs it is still one of the major tasks, they recognize that it is only one of many needs.

"It is not only the child with the illness that needs help," says Edward D. Paradiso, president of the foundation. "The mental and emotional attitudes of the parents are an important ingredient in the patient's success in living with the disease." Moreover, if the family is exclusively preoccupied with the sick child, "nobody has a life," he adds.

Programs are supported to provide counseling of this nature, as well as education, screening, and counseling for family members and others of childbearing age.

The foundation has been co-sponsor with the New York Academy of Sciences of three international conferences on Cooley's Anemia. These events have provided a forum for new ideas to be introduced and old ideas to be reexamined.

On the research front several well-defined problems are being tackled. Now that it is known that most thalassemics produce hemoglobins with too many alpha chains and too few beta chains, scientists are trying to find a way to lower the rate of alpha chain production. Others are exploring the feasibility of performing a transplant of healthy bone marrow to the thalassemic early in life. The relentless search for an agent to remove excess iron goes on. And progress in prenatal diagnosis, for those who want it, is bright.

Finally, on a molecular level, the most recent accomplishment is the synthesis in the laboratory of rabbit hemoglobin DNA from rabbit RNA. What this can mean in the future is that the time may not be too far off when it will no longer be necessary for millions with sickle cell disease and thalassemia to live with an abnormal hemoglobin in their blood.

Is there a future for Susan and Paul? If the present momentum of research in this age-old disorder is maintained, the answer could be yes.

9

Cystic Fibrosis

When Norman starts college in September and makes new friends, he is prepared for some very uncomfortable questions. "Why don't you do something about that cough? How come you eat so much and stay so thin? What are all those pills you keep popping?" He will quickly reassure them that his cough is not contagious. In time he will also explain about cystic fibrosis—a hereditary disorder that afflicts one in every 1,500 newborn babies (mostly white).

Until twenty years ago a child born with cystic fibrosis had a less than 50–50 chance of surviving to school age. Few made it beyond adolescence. Today, thanks to better diagnosis and aggressive treatment, as many as 70 to 80 percent can hope to reach adulthood.

CF is a notorious masquerader. It has been diagnosed as chronic bronchitis, pneumonia, celiac disease, and malnutrition. Norman's first problem in infancy was with food. Although he drained his bottles voraciously, his hunger was never satisfied. Repeated change of formula stopped neither the diarrhea, the crying, nor the failure to gain weight. Matters became worse when he developed a hacking cough that he could not shake.

But between the bouts of discomfort he was a responsive, lovable baby whose grandmother would say when she kissed him, "How can someone as sweet as you taste so salty?"

The underlying problem in CF is in neither the lung, the digestive system, nor the salt on the skin. It is in the inheritance of a double dose of a defective gene controlling the glands that secrete sweat, tears, saliva, and mucus. As in other recessive disorders (Tay-Sachs disease, sickle cell disease, PKU, etc.), it is transmitted when each parent is a carrier and each passes on his defective gene.

There are close to 10,000,000 carriers of the CF gene in the United States—the most common defective gene among white Americans. The probability in each pregnancy, you will recall, is one in four for a baby with both normal genes; one in two for a baby who, like his parents, will not suffer from the disease but will be a carrier; and one in four for a child with CF.

Excessively salty tears and the salty sweat that Norman's grandmother tasted on his skin pose no special problems. (When too much salt is lost in hot weather, it needs to be replaced.) The abnormal mucus, however, is life-threatening. Normal mucus is clear, fluid, and free-flowing and helps clear out germs and dirt from the lungs and air passages. The thick mucus in cystic fibrosis clogs the small bronchial tubes in the lungs, interferes with normal breathing, and, as the blockage persists, infections flourish. Sometimes lungs are permanently damaged.

The mucus also plugs the ducts of the pancreas—the organ that supplies rich digestive enzymes to the small intestine—so that the enzymes cannot get through. This means that food is only partially digested and provides little nutrition. The result is partial starvation in the midst of plenty.

148

Taking care of a boy or girl with CF is a round-the-clock affair with sleepless nights and anxiety-filled days.

The digestive problems are relatively easy to manage. Tablets of pancreatic enzymes taken at meals replace the natural enzymes blocked from reaching the intestine. A low-fat, high-protein diet usually augmented by vitamins supplies the proper nutrition. Norman still eats frequently and consumes large quantities for a young man with such a slight build, but while he sometimes looks longingly at the mounds of french fries his friends devour, it is really no hardship at all to pass them up.

The mucus in the lungs is the major threat, and getting rid of it is far more difficult. One victim describes it as "coaxing the ketchup out of the bottle." Several times a day Norman undergoes "postural drainage." He is placed in a special position determined by the areas of the lungs that need draining. Gentle clapping on his back begins to loosen the mucus, and he can breathe and function again. He hopes that he can now limit the treatments to one before his first class in the morning and another in the evening. He still sleeps in a mist tent where a pump supplies a mist of water particles that help thin the mucus. Some patients continue to take antibiotics every day of their lives; others, more successful in warding off infection, get by with antibiotics only when sporadic infections develop.

Faithful adherence to this demanding regimen enabled Norman to finish high school with honors and to win the biology medal "for the most creative independent project." It is also the regimen that is keeping thousands of young CF children going today. No easier answers are yet in sight.

Because Norman is an only child, his mother's days revolved mainly around the constant care and vigilance his condition required. When asked if the decision to have no more children followed the CF diagnosis, she answered simply, "There was no need to make a decision." By Norman's third birthday the marriage was over. While some parents are drawn closer together by a child with a genetic disorder, even one with severe chronic aspects, it is just as likely to place an intolerable strain on the marriage. Norman's father could not live with the day-to-day reminder of the illness, his role in transmitting the defective gene, and his bad luck in choosing a woman with the same defective gene. Most of all, he could not live with the fear and uncertainty of its happening again with future children.

As yet it is possible to give genetic counseling in CF "only after the fact"—after the birth of an affected child. Physicians now can arrive at a correct diagnosis without difficulty, and there is a growing awareness of the disease among physicians. Some babies born with an intestinal obstruction (meconium ileus) requiring immediate surgery are diagnosed in the first days of life. Diagnosis of the child who develops symptoms later is simple and accurate. A good medical history, plus a test for increased salt content of a small sample of sweat, tell the story.

The parents can now be told, "Each of you is a carrier of the defective gene. Your good gene protects you from the illness, but when each of you purely by chance passes on your defective gene to the baby, he has no such protection. The probability is only one in four, but it happened with Norman. This does not mean that the next three babies will necessarily be normal. The same probability exists in each pregnancy."

They are also told, "We cannot yet offer you a prenatal test on the baby in utero, as we have for other genetic diseases where identification allows you to make a decision about abortion."

Some counseled parents decide not to run the risk again and turn to adoption or artificial insemination or settle for no more children at all. A significant number, however, still take their chances, depending only on faith that the next time the odds will be in their favor. Many have learned that chance has no memory when another CF child is born.

Would parents at risk use a prenatal test if it were available? An impressive number say yes.

It is not only such parents who require a test but also their close relatives, for those who prove to be carriers will need before-the-fact counseling. One in every twenty white Americans is a carrier of the CF gene, and the risk of CF children is obviously greater in a family where the defective gene has already been identified.

Now, after years of disappointing experiences, there is hope that success is at hand for identifying carriers and affected babies in utero. Northwestern University geneticist Dr. Henry Nadler's research implicates an enzyme found in the pancreas, lungs, sweat, saliva, and serum—all sites in the body associated with CF.

Mount Sinai School of Medicine geneticist Dr. Kurt Hirschhorn is now on the track of another enzyme that CF patients lack which may be useful both in detecting carriers and in spotting the disease in the unborn fetus.

Still another provocative clue comes from studies with oysters dredged from the Gulf of Mexico. University of Texas scientists Drs. Barbara Bowman and Don Barnett have isolated three protein substances from CF patients that set off a chain of events in the oyster gills similar to what happens in the respiratory tracts of affected humans. As the fine hairlike cilia in the oyster's gills wave in a rhythmic beat, they move water and other substances through. When serum from normal individuals is applied, the cilia continue to wave. In contrast, CF serum triggers the release of a cloud of mucus from the gills, and within minutes the cilia are bogged down in the thickening exudate. In half an hour they come to a complete halt. The oyster is now an animal model of CF.

The researchers have already demonstrated the same effect with cells grown from the amniotic fluid of a mother known to have the CF gene. Their optimism about a test in the near future is well founded.

What does the future hold for Norman? It is still too early to predict his life-span. An adult generation with CF is too new a phenomenon, but there is every reason to believe that Norman can pursue his dream of becoming a geneticist. He has the ability, and the drive, and as long as he continues to take care of himself, he will have the physical stamina required. Among CF adults today are teachers, graduate students, pharmacists, and computer programmers. Doctors who have treated CF children over the years are impressed with their higher than average intelligence.

For the adult with CF, intellectual prowess alone may not be enough to overcome his handicap. "They don't come right out and say it," a young man describes his job-hunting experiences, "but it's there when they don't hire you. Ignorance and fear can't help matters. . . ." Experience has proved CF adults to be good workers, with absentee records that compare favorably to their healthy colleagues.

Many find it difficult to make the transition from the sheltered climate of the home and family to being responsible for their own care. "How much longer must I sleep in a mist tent?" some ask. Doctors today do not view the tent as a must for all. Too, there are real financial problems which become urgent to those over twenty-one who no longer can call on public funds. Medication and equipment for CF patients alone cost as much as $2,000 a year. Some resent going to a pediatrician or children's clinic for care, even though they cannot find professional know-how on CF elsewhere.

Recognizing the special problems of the young CF adult, the National Cystic Fibrosis Research Foundation, with a national network of 110 research centers and more than 300 chapters and branches, added a Young Adult Services Committee. Doctors, educators, social workers, business people, etc. are available to help the young CF adult with vocational guidance and rehabilitation, to steer him to sources of financial help, and to help him cope with his personal adjustment.

Norman is determined that he will not let CF "rule" him, but he acknowledges that he would be foolish to deny its existence and its impact on his future. Does he plan to marry? Certainly—at the right time and with the right girl. How about children? Until recently infertility among CF males was the general rule. Now several have fathered children.

On this point he is adamant. "Sure I'm glad I was born, but I would not want to bring another CF child into the world. If my wife is a carrier, the risk is too high. Even if she isn't, the best my son or daughter could be is a CF carrier. That too I can't see. Anyway," he chides the interviewer, "do you always ask nineteen-year-old college freshmen about their plans for fatherhood?"

10

*Wilson's Disease
—A Problem of Copper*

If you were to ask Jimmy Carter how it feels to have made medical history, he would be puzzled by the question, for as far back as he can remember he has led a normal healthy life and has little doubt that he will continue to do so. The medication that he takes by mouth every day and the not too restrictive diet he follows impose no special hardship.

"What's so strange," he would counter, "about not eating chocolate, nuts, shellfish, and broccoli?" His friends suffering from acne and allergy have more severe prohibitions.

The fact is that Jimmy will not outgrow his ailment as he would if it were acne. He is a victim of Wilson's disease, a rare genetic disorder that can cripple both mentally and physically and can lead to early death. But Jimmy is probably the first beneficiary of a series of medical discoveries made at the precise moment in history when he needed them most: a test that could detect the disease years before his first symptoms would appear; a medication that when started early enough could prevent its inexorable ravages; a doctor in the right place and at the right time to apply these discoveries, often in the face of discouraging odds.

Wilson's disease is a striking example of how a defective gene interacts with the environment, and the giant strides made in the last two decades in bringing it under control may well serve as a prototype in other genetic disorders.

There had never been a hint of hereditary defects (or for that matter any serious illness) in the Carter family when Mrs. Carter shared the unexpected but not unwelcome news with her three girls that she was pregnant. Their reactions were mixed. "What will my friends say?" from the seventeen-year-old. "Will I have to share my room?" was the concern of the eight-year-old, not prepared to relinquish her position as the youngest in the family. Carol, almost twelve, jumped up from the table, grimaced, and muttered some unintelligible sounds.

"Take the marbles out of your mouth," Mr. Carter admonished her. It was unusual for him to be sharp with Carol, who, although he would not acknowledge it, was somewhat of a favorite. He knew the ways of preteen girls were sometimes strange, but tonight his patience was exhausted. Her antics, it seemed to him, were not just signs of impending adolescence but were more like those of a disintegrating personality.

The next few months brought a mixture of joy and sorrow for the family. Jimmy was born on Thanksgiving—healthy and beautiful. Even the small initial reservations about a new baby were soon dispelled. He was a delightful, responsive, and undemanding child. But Carol got perceptibly worse. Her gait, formerly graceful and springy, was now awkward and shaky; her handwriting, formerly neat and precise, became no better than an illegible scrawl. She occupied a seat in school but was clearly no longer a student. Her teacher was painfully aware of a gaping mouth from which saliva drooled uncontrolled. Worst of all were the frequent and unpredictable episodes of rage and depression. Although she would not admit it, Carol could no longer cope either at school or at home.

Throughout that troubled year Carol had been seen by a number of doctors. None had a clue to the nature of her baffling behavior. The grim climax came in the spring when she started home from school one day but never made it. The awkward gait suddenly turned into a complete paralysis; the mumbled speech silenced into no speech at all. And so the next day instead of a seat in school Carol occupied a bed at the Neurological Institute of the Columbia Presbyterian Hospital.

Three weeks of intensive observations and batteries of tests finally culminated in the news that the stunned Mrs. Carter brought home from the hospital. "We will do our best," the doctors told her gently, "but with Wilson's disease we can promise little." She now had a name for Carol's strange illness, one which she had never heard of until that moment. The poor prognosis was only part of the burden she had to bring back to the family. The incredible fact was that Carol's problem had not started recently. She had been born with it, in fact inherited it from a perfectly healthy mother and father. Mrs. Carter could neither accept nor understand the news. What was unmistakably clear, however, was that if Carol had inherited the defect there was a grave danger that the other children might have as well.

At the time Carol was diagnosed more than forty years had passed since Wilson's disease had been described by the British neurologist whose name it bears and thirty years since its hereditary nature was recognized. Nevertheless, the true nature of the disease eluded doctors. It manifested itself in a variety of ways—in severe liver damage for some, in others, like Carol, such severe neurological damage that normal speech and movement were virtually impossible. Others more acutely affected were even incorrectly labeled psychotic and received needless shock therapy or, worse still, were confined to mental hospitals.

157

Its victims were of varied origin—European, Chinese, Japanese, Malaysian, Eskimo, etc. Some were as young as five when stricken, others over forty. Prognosis—uniformly bad.

No matter what form the disease took, all shared one common characteristic—too much copper in the body, in the wrong places and in excessive amounts. It was not even necessary to look for the copper in Carol with elaborate laboratory tests. She had a greenish ring of copper deposited around the cornea in her eye—the Kayser-Fleischer ring described as far back as 1902 in a patient mistakenly believed to be suffering from multiple sclerosis.

Because we cannot escape taking in copper in our food and drink (including water from copper pipes and whiskey from copper stills) and because a small amount of copper in the body is essential for good health, we have genes that direct the orderly metabolism of the metal. To have a single dose of the defective gene Carol had still allows for normal function. The same genetic rule that applies to carriers of Tay-Sachs disease, thalassemia, sickle cell disease, and other recessive disorders applies to carriers of Wilson's, like Mr. and Mrs. Carter. Inheriting a double dose of the defective gene, one from each parent, means that copper piles up in the nervous system, brain, eye, liver, kidney, etc. It may take from five to forty years for enough copper to accumulate for the disease to show up. For Carol Carter it took twelve. Was there any way of determining if the same process was at work in the other children?

Had this question been asked only a few years back the answer would have been, "We will have to wait and see; there is no way of predicting now who will show signs of the disease in the future." But something new was at hand the day Mrs. Carter asked the question—a recently developed test that promised for the first time to reveal whether any of the other children had also inherited a double dose of the defective gene.

The test was still so new that only a few doctors in the country were familiar with it and only a handful of laboratories were actually performing it. By a most fortunate coincidence the man who discovered the test and was most experienced with it was at that moment working in a laboratory across the street almost close enough for Carol to see from her hospital window.

Dr. I. Herbert Scheinberg had recently accepted an appointment at the New York State Psychiatric Institute, Columbia University. After completing his training at Harvard Medical School, he remained in Boston, where he became interested in Wilson's disease while working at Children's Hospital. Today he is a professor of medicine at the Albert Einstein College of Medicine, Yeshiva University, New York City, and internationally renowned for his continuing contribution to the study of Wilson's disease.

Looking for clues, Dr. Scheinberg turned his attention to a copper-rich protein normally present in blood—ceruloplasmin (named for its blue color by the two Swedish chemists who had first described it only a few years earlier).

With increased copper in the eyes, liver, brain, etc. of Wilson's disease victims, was it possible, Dr. Scheinberg speculated, that this copper-rich substance in the blood (it could be measured) was also increased? Repeated tests revealed that ceruloplasmin levels were indeed changed but much to his surprise, not, as he expected, increased but diminished to imperceptible levels. He had no explanation for this curious phenomenon, but he did have a test not only for those who were already sick and not yet diagnosed, but also for brothers and sisters who had not manifested any symptoms but might well be vulnerable.

"Most crucial," says Dr. Scheinberg, "is testing younger sisters and brothers because when more than one member of the family succumbs, it is generally at about the same age."

Carol's older sister, still healthy at eighteen, was probably safe, but for her younger sister and baby brother, Jimmy, the information was vital.

Within the next few days Dr. Scheinberg tested all the children. The older sister, as had been expected, was normal, as was the younger sister. But Jimmy had the same deficiency of ceruloplasmin as did Carol. He too had inherited two defective genes. And although no outward signs were evident, he was slowly accumulating excess copper in his vital organs that would in ten or twelve years inevitably subject him to the catastrophic events suffered by Carol.

For Dr. Scheinberg defining the problem was easier than providing the solutions. First, both Carol and Jimmy needed from that moment on to be spared taking in any food or drink that would add to the copper deposits—hence the diet with no shellfish, chocolate, nuts, etc. An unpalatable resin helpful in removing some of the copper in food was added to their diets.

Removing the copper already piled up in vital organs was not so simple. Even Jimmy, still without symptoms, had an increased copper level in his liver dating back probably to the days in his mother's womb. The best remedy available at the time was a substance developed in England during World War I as an antidote to arsenic—a threat in poison gas warfare. BAL (British anti-Lewisite) was never used for its original purpose, but it was learned that it was also effective against other heavy metals including lead, mercury, and copper. Used for the first time for Wilson's disease patients in 1951, BAL produced remarkable improvement.

BAL allowed Carol to return to school, although she was far from normal. And BAL had serious drawbacks—it was a harsh substance, effective only by painful injection. Despite Carol's improvement, there were many days of uncertainty and anxiety for the Carters. They were saved from total despair by the ever-present hope that something better than BAL would soon come along, not only to keep Carol going but also gentle enough to be given to Jimmy, still a healthy and thriving child.

The news for which the family waited so eagerly finally came

160

through when they arrived for a periodic checkup in 1956. A doctor from Cambridge, England, Dr. John M. Walshe, had discovered a new medication that promised to accomplish even more than BAL but without any of its harsh side effects. Most appealing was that it could be taken by mouth.

Like Dr. Scheinberg, Dr. Walshe was working in Boston in the early 1950's. At that time he was studying patients with liver disease, attempting to find out which amino acids they were excreting in the urine. Using paper chromatography, a technique where each amino acid leaves its telltale spot on a test paper, he noted an unfamiliar spot recovered from the urine of four of the patients. Checking back he learned that all four were receiving penicillin treatment for one reason or another. The new spot was an amino acid hitherto not identified in human body fluids— penicillamine, a substance closely related to penicillin but without its antibiotic powers. Most provocative to him was its structure that should have made it very active chemically.

Meanwhile, he, like Dr. Scheinberg, had become interested in Wilson's disease while in Boston, and so when he returned to Cambridge, England, he decided to put the reactive chemical to work in the body, hoping that it would bind to the copper in the tissues of Wilson's disease patients.

It worked! His first patient, completely bedridden when he began treating her, is now leading a normal married life. For the Carter family on the other side of the ocean the substance was to mean new hope and comfort for Carol and a preventive medication for Jimmy, gentle and safe enough for a baby.

Jimmy is now finished with high school and, as Dr. Scheinberg wrote the author in 1972, "continues to do beautifully with respect to his Wilson's disease. He remains completely asymptomatic and takes his medication with reasonable faithfulness."

Carol too made beautiful progress on the new therapy. She returned to school, earned a high school diploma, and found a job in a local store within a few months. However, her nervous system

161

and other organs in her body had already suffered extensive damage which even the new medication could not reverse completely.

Jimmy made medical history in growing from infancy to adulthood on a regimen that thwarted a hitherto-hopeless illness. Since Dr. Walshe's first patient, scores of others have been saved. The key to survival is correct and early diagnosis and the immediate adoption of a program that combines diet and medication. So far penicillamine is still the best medication available.

A little-known crisis arose with penicillamine after Jimmy and Carol had been on it for a few years and doing well. Happily for them it was resolved before they knew about it. Because penicillamine was costly to produce and because there was such a limited use for it, the company that was supplying it considered not making it any longer. Dismayed at the consequences for patients who were uniquely dependent on it, Dr. Scheinberg pleaded with the company not to cut off the supply. A leading Midwestern newspaper opened its pages to the cause. The company yielded; the availability of penicillamine continued without interruption.

There have been some unexpected bonuses, for since that time penicillamine has proved to be effective in the management of another unrelated genetic disease—cystinuria. The latest chapter in the drug's role in health and disease is still being written, again in an unrelated disorder but one that is by no means rare—rheumatoid arthritis.

Several years ago New York internist Dr. Israeli A. Jaffe observed that when he treated rheumatoid arthritis patients with penicillamine there was noticeable improvement in both the biochemical tests associated with the disease and, more important, the patient's clinical condition. Subsequent reports confirmed the early observations. There was no explanation for how it worked, but the results were sufficiently encouraging to widen its use.

162

Wilson's Disease—A Problem of Copper

It has just come through a five-year trial in five medical centers in Britain. Only patients with severe rheumatoid arthritis were selected; some received the drug, others a placebo. The results were published in *The Lancet* in 1973. Judging by the clinical condition of the patients and laboratory tests, penicillamine was significantly superior to the placebo. The data convinced the British Committee on the Safety of Medicines to approve the use of penicillamine in severe rheumatoid arthritis. (It still awaits similar approval from the FDA in the United States.) Meanwhile, tests continue in Britain. Less severe arthritics will now be tested, and in addition, a comparison will be made between the effectiveness of penicillamine and a very old treatment—gold salts.

It may well be that the spin-offs of Dr. Walshe's discovery can ultimately be more far-reaching than he ever dreamed when he introduced it and when Dr. Scheinberg fought to keep it on the market a few years later.

Thanks to better diagnosis (methods yielding more accurate results than ceruloplasmin level alone have since been devised) and availability of effective medication, Wilson's disease is no longer considered a progressive and fatal disease as it was when Jimmy was born. Identifying the victim when another member of the family has already been found is routine today. Not so smooth is the correct diagnosis when the disease strikes a family for the first time.

Doctors are becoming alert to the strange guises this rare disorder takes. Among children and young adults chronic liver disease may be the clue. Dr. Scheinberg and his colleague Dr. Irmin Sternlieb cite the experience of seven such patients who were treated for up to four and a half years before the true nature of the illness was discovered. Until neurological symptoms developed, there was no reason for the doctors to suspect that there was more than liver disease to be looked for. Treatment with penicillamine despite the delay eliminated most of the symptoms of the

163

disease in all except one. "The course of these patients," they advise "is our reason for recommending strongly that in every young patient with chronic hepatitis, Wilson's disease should be considered and the diagnosis ruled out or confirmed."

Even more compelling of recognition are the victims who exhibit psychiatric or neurotic behavior as a first symptom. In fact, fully one-third of all Wilson's disease victims come to a physician's attention for precisely these reasons. A report from the Mayo Clinic describes the improvement scored by a number of such individuals after treatment. Comprehension, recall, and memory were consistently improved. IQ scores were raised. Not only were the early gains retained, but improvement continued after five to six years of treatment.

Early diagnosis in children is particularly crucial. Youngsters started on treatment under the age of twelve were spared the emotional and intellectual disturbances that afflict more than 50 percent who, like Carol, remain untreated. "Because of the therapeutic effectiveness of decoppering . . ." suggests Dr. Scheinberg, "diagnostic tests for Wilson's disease should be applied to all mentally ill who seek medical care."

A new generation of individuals with Wilson's disease are, like Jimmy, reaching adulthood, contemplating marriage and parenthood. What are the risks in raising a family? With the disorder such a rarity, the probability is very small that he will marry a carrier. Nevertheless, it is estimated that there are 400,000 carriers in the United States. There may also be a larger concentration in some ethnic groups and geographical locations, as was shown by the classical contribution to the genetic pattern of the disease made by Professor Alexander G. Bearn, Cornell University Medical College. In the New York area two main groups had the highest incidence—Jews from Eastern Europe and non-Jews from the Mediterranean regions, especially Sicily.

Healthy sisters and brothers need to know if they are carriers. A research team headed by Dr. Sternlieb developed a method to detect carriers. With this information, it is now possible to predict the risks, which are similar to that in other recessive genetic disorders described elsewhere in the book (Tay-Sachs disease, thalassemia, sickle cell disease, etc.).

The Carter family is a good illustration that "chance has no memory" and that the same risk exists in every pregnancy when both parents are carriers: one in four for a child with two normal genes; two in four for a child with one defective gene (a carrier); one in four for a child with a double dose of the defective gene (a child with Wilson's disease). The often misunderstood statement that one-quarter will be normal, one-half will be carriers, and one-quarter will be affected applies only to thousands and thousands of births. Such statistics cannot be applied to a single family. Such an erroneous impression would have lulled the Carters into believing that with Carol's diagnosis made, it could not happen to them again.

Prenatal diagnosis is not yet possible, but the knowledge and understanding of the risks involved make possible more informed decisions.

Information comes to interested families from varied sources. Several years ago a family was referred to Dr. Scheinberg to confirm the diagnosis in one child with symptoms and to test the other children still free of symptoms. The referral was made by a physician in Philadelphia after an anxious mother consulted her eye doctor. "Please examine my daughter for Wilson's disease" was her plea to the startled doctor. When he learned that there was no history of the disorder in the family, he was even more puzzled at the mother's specific request. Much to his surprise he soon found the single most characteristic diagnostic sign of Wilson's disease in the child's eyes—the green gold Kayser-Fleischer ring around the cornea. This was precisely what the mother herself had seen that had aroused her suspicions. He lost no time in sending the whole family to Dr. Scheinberg for consultation.

In a summary sent along was included the note that "the mother had apparently taken the youngster to the ophthalmologist after reading an article in a women's journal concerning Wilson's disease." * Dr. Scheinbert instituted intensive treatment, the best promise for the best prognosis, at once.

* "Inborn Errors of Metabolism" by Augusta Greenblatt. *Family Circle* magazine, April, 1967.

11

*Inborn Errors**
—Detectable and Correctable

PKU—Phenylketonuria

Maureen has always considered herself lucky—in school, where she made many good friends; her first job, where she met Sean; and the year her first child was born. "If it had been 1950 instead of 1970," she says, "Kitty would probably be a hopelessly retarded, unhappy, agitated little girl—maybe doomed to die an early death in an institution."

Kitty is a victim of a rare inherited inborn error of metabolism: PKU—phenylketonuria. She is among the 1 in 20,000 babies born every year who, owing to a double dose of a defective gene, cannot metabolize phenylalanine, an amino acid found in milk and other

---

* In a sense all inherited diseases are "inborn errors," but scientists use the term in a narrower context to describe a disorder in which a mutation of a single gene results in a specific abnormal enzyme or other protein. The "errors" described in this chapter share one characteristic—*one* step in a series of chemical reactions needed for good health is disrupted by the deviant gene.

protein foods. When the phenylalanine piles up in the body, the consequences are brain damage, hyperactive and sometimes destructive behavior, and death for some in childhood. A smaller number survive to early adulthood.

Because he cannot metabolize an amino acid involved in making the pigments in hair, eyes, and skin, the phenylketonuric is often blond, fair-skinned and blue-eyed. In a family where other members are dark-skinned, the child with the disorder is markedly lighter.

When PKU is diagnosed early in infancy before the protein in regular milk has had a chance to do its harm, and a special formula substituted at once, the bleak picture changes. Kitty was identified as a PKU child when she was four days old. From that moment on she was rigidly restricted in her nonprotein diet and is, at four, a seemingly normal little girl—mentally, physically, and in her behavior.

Maureen appreciates what could have been. A first cousin, who was born in 1950, when the practice of looking for PKU in all infants was not yet a reality, was four years old before his condition was recognized. She recalls him vividly. Her last memory was a visit to the hospital before he died at sixteen.

PKU was first described in 1934 by Norwegian physician and biochemist Dr. Asborg Folling. A distraught mother came to him for help for her two children—both severely retarded and extremely hard to manage. Like the other doctors who had seen the children earlier, there was little help Dr. Folling could give.

He was particularly puzzled however by what he found in a routine test of their urine. When he added the simple chemical ferric chloride, the urine turned a deep blue-green. Was there a link between the blue-green color and the mental retardation? He tested additional retarded children. Ten showed the same reaction. The color was due to a substance called phenylpyruvic acid; the condition is PKU.

Maureeen and Sean are both carriers of the defective gene, and they now know that the risk in every future pregnancy is one in four for another PKU child.

Dr. Folling's discovery not only was the first solid link between biochemistry and mental function but also launched a new era in the detection of genetic disorders. PKU is the first inborn error of metabolism for which mass screening of newborn is suitable and is now one of almost a dozen disorders screened for in millions of babies yearly.* In each instance prompt and vigorous action can avert disaster.

In the days before the underlying basis of the disorder was established, a variety of remedies was tried—hormones, vitamins, minerals, etc. All were futile. What was needed was not something added but something taken away.

The basis of Kitty's successful diet is a powdered extract of protein from which the harmful amino acid phenylalinine has been removed. When mixed with water, it becomes a substitute for the meat, milk, cheese, nuts, and poultry that she would otherwise be eating. Fruits and vegetables with low-protein content, including apples, bananas, carrots, celery, pineapple, strawberries, tomatoes, and watermelon, are allowed in limited quantities.

It is not an easy diet to prepare or to adhere to. Not every patient does well on a diet so poor in protein, and many suffer poor growth. But the alternative, PKU, is clearly worse. The first patient who received the diet showed a reversal of all biochemical abnormalities. His behavior improved; his blond hair quickly darkened. The metabolic block was successfully broken. Very young children, in whom brain damage was not yet far advanced, improved mentally, but older victims remained retarded.

Another problem is that by the age of six or seven it becomes increasingly difficult to enforce a rigid diet on some children. Kitty accepted the diet well. She has never known any other and

* Today screening for PKU is compulsory in forty-eight states in the United States and voluntary in two. Similar programs have also been instituted in Canada and Europe.

has no sisters or brothers whose more attractive meals could tempt her. She may, however, by the time she reaches school age begin to balk. Happily she may be permitted some relaxation in the rigidity without sliding back. Doctors believe that she will continue to maintain the level of intelligence she has already achieved.

PKU has been found in diverse ethnic groups including Japanese, Arabs, and Armenians. It is noticeably absent among Ashkenazi Jews, both in the United States and Israel, and among blacks. In fact, after three years of screening in Washington, D.C., where most of the births are to black families, the program was discontinued when not a single positive was found. The highest incidence of PKU is among nothern Europeans, particularly the Irish and other Celts. Among them it is usually estimated at 1 in 20,000 but may be higher in some geographic areas. Massachusetts, with the oldest statewide screening program in the country, has tested almost 1,000,000 babies since 1963. By 1973, 67 (1 in 15,000) with typical PKU and 57 (1 in 17,000) with atypical PKU had been discovered.

A new generation of PKU victims has reached adulthood free of many of the handicaps they would have endured in the past. Many have married and have had children. There is increasing evidence that among more than 90 children born to PKU mothers almost all showed some type of defect, including mental retardation, raising the specter that long-term therapy may produce more retardation than it will prevent.

Genetic counseling in PKU families, to be meaningful, must provide not only a clear understanding of what can be done to provide a healthy life for the PKU child, but a view as well of the difficulties and unsolved problems. While there is a test for carriers that can identify the trait in sisters, brothers, and other relatives, there is as yet no prenatal test to identify PKU in utero. An extra edge, it is believed, can be given to the unborn baby of a PKU mother if she restricts her diet in pregnancy.

Despite the dilemmas, problems, and occasional controversies about the wisdom of the PKU screening and treatment programs, the prevailing view today is that it is worthwhile—both to a society relieved of the burden of care required in the past and to the individual and family spared a retarded child.

Indeed, so gratifying has been the outcome that, in the opinion of Yale's Dr. Leon E. Rosenberg and McGill's Dr. Charles Scriver, "It is possible that the mentally retarded with eczema, pigment dilution and seizures will become a historical oddity to be found as a description in old text books, but almost never encountered in the practice of today's medicine."

MSUD (Maple Syrup Urine Disease)

To many New Englanders the aroma of maple syrup is associated with crisp wintry days and the rich sap flowing from tapped trees. To one New England mother, however, it was an odor on her baby's diaper which she had tragically learned from past experience signaled rapid deterioration and early death.

So it had been for four of her children. Each was normal at birth, but within the first week of life the scent of maple syrup was detected in the urine, and then the child's appetite waned, he became lethargic, sickened, and died. One lived to be three months; three died before they were two weeks old.

At the time biochemical studies failed to reveal the basis for the strange odor and the fatal course associated with it. But Boston's Dr. J. A. Menkes and his colleagues knew they were dealing with a distinct and hitherto unrecognized genetic disorder. They reported their observations in *Pediatrics* in 1954.

By 1959 two research teams in the United States and Britain independently confirmed that it was an inborn error of metabolism and identified the error. In MSUD there is an accumulation in the blood of three amino acids, with some of the excess spilling

171

over into the urine. The fact is that the amino acids leucine, isoleucine, and valine in appropriate amounts are essential to good health, both mental and physical.

In MSUD a deficient enzyme disrupts the metabolism of these amino acids, causing the buildup and production of abnormal products. Like PKU, the disease occurs when a child inherits a double dose of the defective gene responsible for that enzyme. (With the precise amino acids identified, the more scientific name-branched chain ketoaciduria [BCKA] has been suggested, but the maple syrup label persists.)

Taking a cue from success with PKU, doctors turned to a similar diet, this time very low in the three offending amino acids implicated in MSUD. Like the PKU diet, it is difficult and expensive, must be started in the first week of life and maintained for a still-undetermined number of years, but it promises to work. At least one little girl continues to function well mentally and physically after six and a half years. Without it, if she had survived at all, it would have been as a severely retarded and sick child.

By 1972, 50 cases from various parts of the world had been identified. Five were found among more than 750,000 newborns screened in Massachusetts, and 2 among 190,000 screened in New York City. Considering the rarity of the disorder, most doctors will probably never encounter it in their professional life, but for the one who does, the odor of maple syrup on a diaper may alert him to a dramatic opportunity to save a life. For doctors in parts of the world where maple syrup is unfamiliar, there is a reminder in the medical literature that "maple syrup smells like burnt sugar."

For the rare family at risk for the disease, a prenatal test is now available. At least two MSUD babies have been identified in utero. At least two mothers need not fear the odor of maple syrup.

Galactosemia

Back in 1908 a doctor reported in a Viennese medical journal of his unusual decision to remove milk from the diet of a sick baby in his care, and substitute in its place "tea with gruel of corn flour." What prompted him was his discovery of an abnormal sugar galactose in the child's urine. Its source was milk, and it should have been metabolized in the body instead of being passed out in the urine.

That was the same year that Dr. Garrod in London (see Chapter 1) delivered his historic Croonian lecture on four "Inborn Errors of Metabolism." Neither he nor the Viennese Dr. von Reuss knew it at the time, but the baby with the milk problem made it five.

Almost thirty years were to pass before galactosemia was to be recognized as a distinct clinical entity characterized by failure to thrive, liver damage, early cataracts, and mental retardation. Almost twenty years more were to pass before the biochemical basis was explained: a deficiency of an enzyme required to metabolize lactose—the chief sugar in milk. Lactose cannot be utilized directly by the cells and tissues. It must first be broken down to glucose. A number of enzymes make this possible; first the lactose is broken down to glucose and galactose, and then the galactose is converted to glucose. Normally the conversion proceeds at a relatively rapid rate, but in the absence or deficiency of the appropriate enzyme, galactose accumulates in the blood and spills over into the urine.

The consequences are varied—ranging from very minor gastrointestinal irritability to the textbook picture of classic galactosemia of liver damage, cataracts, and mental retardation.

Today galactosemia joins inherited disorders like PKU, MSUD, Wilson's disease, and others that, when identified early enough, can be successfully treated by limiting the offending substance—in this instance, milk.

173

Some galactosemics develop the capacity to handle milk and milk products despite the faulty enzyme production with which they are born. They grow normally, free of most of the ravages of galactosemia except for an increased risk of cataracts at an early age. Indeed, a number of asymptomatic cases have been found only when they have participated in family genetic studies (not unlike the occasional sickle-cell disease victim similarly identified).

The knowledge about galactosemia today has all the ingredients for successful genetic counseling and management. The mode of transmission is understood—inheritance of a double dose of the defective gene. The faulty enzyme has been identified. There is a spot test suitable for mass screening of newborns, and prenatal testing to detect the disorder in utero when a risk is suspected is also available, and there is a diet that can reduce the damage of the disorder to virtually zero.

Because the diet gives the galactosemic child an optimistic future and also because for some the disease itself may be minor (IQ as high as 124 has been found), Dr. Henry Nadler, who in 1969 developed the prenatal test, questions the necessity of using it at all. He does advise the mother who has already had one galactosemic child to eliminate milk from her diet during pregnancy, thus creating a safer climate for her unborn baby in utero.

Mass screening of newborns continues to turn up unsuspected cases. By 1973 the Massachusetts program found 5 among more than 500,000 screened (an incidence of 1 in 110,000), and a New York state program yielded an incidence of 1 in 35,000 live births.

Prompt removal of milk from the baby's diet with continued vigilance as the child grows older are the keys to a healthy future.

Galactokinase Deficiency

In contrast with classic galactosemia, which usually makes its presence known in the first few months of life, there is another defect of galactose metabolism much more insidious but fortunately with just a single serious effect—cataracts at an early age. Indeed, because of the absence of other symptoms, the condition may be unrecognized. Unlike cataracts caused by aging, injury, and other metabolic disorders, these cataracts are completely avoidable on a milk-restricted diet. In some instances cataracts that have already started to develop begin to regress after the diet is instituted.

A 1965 report in *The Lancet* described a forty-four-year-old man who had developed cataracts at the age of nine. (His sisters now in their sixties had also developed cataracts at the ages of five and seven.) Like the classic galactosemic, he excreted galactose in the urine, but he was mentally normal and was otherwise in good health.

With identification of additional victims in the next few years this newly discovered cause of juvenile cataracts was nailed down as still another inborn error of metabolism, transmitted by two defective genes by carrier parents. The deficient enzyme is galactokinase. The victim cannot handle milk and milk products properly.

Unlike other recessive disorders, in which the carrier's (heterozygote) biggest problem is transmitting the defective gene to his offspring, he himself, with the single defective gene, is also at increased risk for early cataracts. While he will not develop the eye disorder in childhood, as the homozygote does, he may well be a victim before the age of forty.

Dr. Ernest Beutler, City of Hope Medical Center, Duarte, California, with the help of a team from the University of Chicago and the National Genetics Foundation in New York, has examined 162 individuals under the age of forty with "unknown" cause of cataracts. The evidence is very strong that reduced galactokinase level is part of the "unknown" cause.

In an appeal to doctors to help locate those at risk, Dr. Beutler asks them to send samples of blood for testing—airmail, special delivery. He promises to perform the tests promptly and report the results promptly.

In October, 1972, a report in *Science* by University of Pennsylvania Dr. Thomas A. Tedesco revealed that the carrier state among blacks may be significantly higher than among whites, placing them at greater risk for premature cataracts when large quantities of milk and milk products are consumed.

A galactose-free diet for those who are totally deficient in galactokinase and a galactose-restricted diet for those with partial impairment can be a significant step in preventive medicine.*

Milk Intolerance

While probably no more than 1 in every 40,000 babies will be born with galactokinase deficiency and 1 in every 35,000 with transferase deficiency (classic galactosemia), there are probably several million children suffering from another milk enzyme deficiency, an enzyme found in the digestive system—lactase. Worldwide intolerance of milk sugar is widespread, with blacks and Orientals affected in largest numbers.

At birth, every baby, regardless of ethnic origin, is endowed with a very high level of lactase, essential to metabolize the food that nature intended for the mainstay of his diet in infancy—milk. With maturity the enzyme level falls, but for some still unexplained reason a substantial number of children experience a greater decline than other children do. By the time they reach school age the same quantity of milk that helped them thrive and grow in their early years can now cause abdominal pain, a feeling of fullness, and diarrhea.

A Johns Hopkins research team reported at the 1971 American Public Health Association Annual Meeting that in Baltimore 58 percent of the black children and 18 percent of the white children in two schools could not tolerate milk. This phenomenon had

* A list of approved foods for those who must limit lactose intake can be found in "Nutritional Therapy of Galactosemia," Dr. R. Koch, *Clinical Pediatrics*, Vol. 4, 571 (1965).

been recognized in non-white adults for a long time, but it was the first evidence that children too were susceptible.

"Since most of the world's population and in particular millions of its hungry and malnourished have varying degrees of lactase deficiency," comments the U.S. government publication *Agricultural Research,* "the problem must be reckoned with. The answer is not, according to the United Nations Protein Advisory Group, to eliminate milk as a protein source in large scale feeding programs for the malnourished. The answer is rather in developing dairy products in which most of the lactose has been predigested and so can be tolerated by all."

Research is now in progress in government laboratories in Philadelphia, Berkeley, and Washington. By June, 1973, some of the treated products included fluid and powdered milk and ice cream with as much as 90 percent of the lactose predigested. There is an added bonus—an enhancement of natural sweetness that diminishes the need for added sugar. Several industrial firms to whom samples were sent expressed interest in them.

Should the early pilot plant success prove to be feasible for large-scale production the day may not be far off when every individual in the world who can benefit from the nutrition of milk need no longer be deprived of it.

Vitamin Dependent Deficiencies

In contrast with genetic disorders than can be treated by removing something from the diet that cannot be managed (such as copper in Wilson's disease, milk and milk products in galactosemia, proteins in PKU and MSUD), there are situations where good health can be restored by *adding* an appropriate substance.

In 1968 a baby was brought to the Yale-New Haven Hospital who at eight months was markedly underweight and mentally retarded. Several other such children had already been observed.

177

One clue to their problem was the presence in the urine of large amounts of a substance called methyl malonic acid, which by coincidence is also found in pernicious anemia—a disease marked by a deficiency of vitamin B_{12}. But the child had normal levels of vitamin B_{12} and, moreover, showed no signs of pernicious anemia.

Quick action in treating the baby was a must if the baby were to be spared further deterioration. Within a few months Dr. Leon Rosenberg succeeded in pinpointing the precise sequence of biochemical events that lead to the disorder. A normal enzyme system is present but fails to function. Vitamin B_{12}, in massive doses (1,000 times the usual amount), activates the system.

After a year of treatment the baby had a normal weight, and his IQ (tested by responses to stimuli etc.) was *100*.

For the most part vitamin-dependent disorders, like other inborn errors of metabolism, are inherited as a double dose of a defective gene from both parents who are carriers (recessive). One notable exception to the hereditary pattern is vitamin D resistant rickets. (Rickets caused by vitamin D deficiency in the diet has virtually disappeared from the American scene.)

In the genetic type, while there is adequate vitamin D in the diet, as well as in the blood and in the cells, it fails to perform its task of activating the protein that will transport calcium from the intestinal tract into the bones. The outcome is poor bone growth with short stature and sometimes crippling. The cure is ingestion of vitamin D * in quantities far beyond the usual requirements.

The defective gene for vitamin D resistant rickets is on the X chromosome, and a single dose transmits the disease, which is dominant. An affected mother can transmit the defect to both sons and daughters with a 50 percent risk in each pregnancy. An affected father who provides his X chromosome to all his

* For the normal child or adult such excessive doses of vitamin can be harmful.

daughters will have only affected daughters. His sons who receive only his Y chromosomes are of course free of the disease.

Where there is a family history of the disorder, genetic counseling can alert the parents to the risk of another affected child. Early detection can alert the doctor to institute vigorous measures with replacement of vitamin D plus other medications that promise to halt the crippling of rickets and other bone deformities.

Addressing himself to the practicing physician who may find genetic diseases depressing because of the limitation of what he can accomplish, Dr. Rosenberg emphasizes that "the vitamin dependent genetic disorders constitute a rather cheering contrast . . . *all* of *them are wholly correctable.*"

At the present time, inborn errors still not correctable far outnumber those that are. Meanwhile, the ongoing search for victims who *can* be treated goes on. Legislation has been drafted for the New York State Senate mandating screening for seven diseases all serious when not detected in time, and all except one (SS) completely preventable.

The promise is that for the taxpayer there will be substantial savings in the staggering sums now spent on long-term institutional care for victims. For parents, such as Maureen and Sean, there is no price tag they can put on keeping Kitty healthy.

12

IQ—Are You Born to Be Smart or Stupid?

You are a high school senior and you are told your IQ is 97. Would you:

1. Withdraw the college applications you have filed?
2. Apply to college because you have always wanted to be an engineer, with hopes of a graduate degree?
3. Offer yourself for sterilization and a bounty of $3,000?

Sound foolish? No more foolish than some of the "serious" talk about IQ (intelligence quotient) on national TV, in newspaper articles, and on college campuses.

Pushing a plea for sterilization with a bounty of $1,000 for each point an IQ fails below 100, is Stanford University's Dr. William B. Shockley (he shared a Nobel Prize for his work with transistors, but admits he is a layman in his studies of IQ). Dr. Shockley believes low IQ is hereditary.

While few are ready to accept Dr. Shockley's proposal on how to protect man's genetic future, he does find an audience for another of his concepts. Dr. Shockley believes that blacks in the United States are genetically inferior as measured by IQ scores and that their depressed socioeconomic status in our society can be attributed to some degree to this inherited inferiority.

Does an IQ of 97 doom you to a menial job? A 1955 study of eighty-nine men who earned PhD degrees in physics, chemistry, and engineering at Ohio State University, University of California (Berkeley), and Cornell revealed that 3 scored between *96* and *100* in IQ tests in high school.

Perhaps no aspect of the question of how much heredity controls the fate of an individual has stirred as much controversy as IQ—intelligence quotient.

IQ, the name and the concept, dates back to the early part of the century to about the same time that scientists were beginning to look for links between heredity and behavior. It was, however, entirely unrelated to heredity at the time. The French government asked psychologist Alfred Binet to devise a test that could identify those students capable of learning in regular public schools and those who needed special schooling. In 1905 he and his collaborator Théodore Simon published the Binet-Simon test—an instrument designed to predict future success in school.

Had Binet chosen a better word than "native intelligence" and claimed instead that he was measuring "academic readiness," he would have been closer to the mark and possibly averted some of the confusion of later years.

Over the years, IQ has come to be endowed with almost mystical powers. Some of the myths that surround it are: It is determined *solely* by heredity and fixed in the genes at conception; it is impervious to change; it is a major factor determining one's success in occupation and status in life; it can be used to categorize ethnic and racial groups; it actually measures that still-to-be-defined quality intelligence.

Dr. Binet arrived at his yardstick of "intelligence" by testing 100 ten-year-olds. Their scores ran the gamut from a four-year-old at one extreme to a fourteen-year-old at the other. The ten-year-old who scored on the four-year level was described as having a mental age of four, the one who scored at the four-teen-year-old level a mental age of fourteen. Since both had a chronological age of ten, a convenient formula was adopted to describe their status. By dividing the mental age by chronological age and multiplying by 100, the IQ was arrived at.

An IQ of 100 means that half of a certain population tests below that score and half tests above it. The range of 90–110 is considered average, 80–90 dull, 70–80 borderline, and below 70 retarded. At the other end of the scale usually over 130 is in the gifted range. (It can be expected that 70 percent of all people tested will have IQ's between 85 and 115, 5 percent below 70, and 5 percent above 130. For the mathematically minded this is a standard deviation of 15 points.) Where is the genius? With so many other factors needed to define a genius few would dare to reduce it to a number.

The tests soon won international acclaim. In the United States the results were as gratifying as Binet had found them in France. They predicted not only success in school, but also in the number of grades completed. In recent years there have been attempts to improve the tests by breaking down various components of intel-lectual function—verbal, reasoning, memory, spatial ability, etc.

In each instance the goal has been to structure a test that will truly reflect innate intelligence unbiased by cultural experience and background. The *consensus of most psychologists, including strong advocates of IQ testing, is that no test to date has succeeded.*

Scores are based on solutions to brief problems and responses to simple questions. Correct answers often depend on verbal ability and attitudes acquired at a given age—clearly the sum of both innate ability and experience. There is still no precise definition of intelligence. The geneticist frustrated at the failure to arrive at an acceptable definition suggests that "intelligence is what is meas-ured by IQ."

While Binet's test was standardized against a relatively homogeneous French population, the challenge in the United States, with its greater ethnic, cultural, social, and economic diversity, was far more complex. Nevertheless, the major IQ tests in use in the United States today have been standardized against native-born white children. Such was the procedure with the first United States version—the Stanford-Binet in 1916—and so it has persisted with the more recent Wechsler Intelligence Scale for Children (WISC), Peabody Picture Vocabulary, and others.

It was not long before IQ testers observed a significant correlation of scores among members of families—the closer the relationship, the stronger was the correlation. Thus identical twins, with the same genetic endowment, had strikingly similar IQ's. Brothers and sisters and nonidentical twins also had a high correlation but not as high as the first group. The IQ scores of children also correlated well with those of their parents.

Evidence pointed toward a hereditary factor, notwithstanding the fact these individuals also shared a very similar environment. How much is biologically determined (in the genes) and how much reflects the environment and culture? One of the earliest answers comes from a landmark work published in 1937: *Twins: A Study of Heredity and Environment.*

Drs. H. H. Newman, F. N. Freeman, and K. J. Holzinger studied 100 pairs of twins—50 identical and 50 same sex fraternal—all of whom lived and were brought up by their parents in the same household. Later they located 19 pairs of identical twins who had been separated before their first birthday, reared apart by different families, some in different towns.

The IQ tests of the two groups do not tell the same story. In contrast with the twins brought up together, whose correlation was 0.91 (1.0 is theoretically the closest), the separated 19 showed a correlation of 0.67. Some differed by as much as 24 IQ points although, even among the separated twins, the cultural differences were not great—all were brought up by white middle-class families.

184

More recently (1966) Sir Cyril Burt, a strong advocate of the influence of heredity, published his studies on 53 pairs of identical twins separated before the age of six months. As expected, they showed a high correlation of IQ but not as high as if they had been reared together. Of greater significance, however, was their school achievement, where the correlation was surprisingly low.

Most revealing was what Sir Cyril found among unrelated children whose IQ showed little correlation but who were reared together. Their achievements in school were surprisingly similar. Indeed, the correlation was as high as that of identical twins reared apart. Clearly IQ alone is not an entirely reliable predictor of success in school. Family, home, school, and community—all add up to make the crucial difference.

Adopted children have been found to have IQ's as much as 20 points higher than those of their biological parents, a fact presumably reflecting the more favorable climate for intellectual growth provided by the adopted family.

When does the environment begin to influence IQ? Long before birth, while the baby is still in utero, say Drs. S. Gorham Babson and David S. Phillips of the University of Oregon Medical School. While it has been known for some time that babies born weighing less than five-and-a-half pounds often show deficits both mentally and physically in their growing years, more precise data were required before it was possible to assess the effect of unfavorable uterine life. Drs. Babson and Phillips found some of the answers in a study reported in the *New England Journal of Medicine,* in November, 1973.

They studied nine pairs of identical twins who differed in birth weight by an average of 36 percent. Of the eight pairs they followed to maturity (eighteen years), the twin that was smaller at birth remained smaller in height and weight. Moreover, their IQ, as tested by three different standardized tests, revealed a consistent difference between the larger and smaller of the pair. In each instance the twin who was larger at birth scored higher on the IQ test, with the gap widening as the children grew older. Interestingly enough, while the larger twin did better on standardized tests than the smaller, among three sets, the smaller twin racked up a higher grade point average in high school. When the parents of these three sets of twins were asked to describe their personalities, it turned out that the smaller twin made a greater effort to achieve, while the larger twin was on the whole "more easy going and self-assured." Here is a clear suggestion of what motivation and drive can accomplish to compensate for a less distinguished IQ related to the unfavorable environmental factor of lower birth weight.

But that handicap is nowhere near as threatening as an infancy and early childhood spent in a materially and intellectually impoverished environment.

Is it possible to compensate for that greater handicap by giving intensive and sustained help very early in life? Many educators and psychologists have long believed this to be possible, but too often their belief was based more on an act of faith than on concrete results. A group at the University of Wisconsin, under the leadership of Professor R. Heber, now has hard data from five years of experience with a bold experiment in a slum area in Milwaukee. Their experiences are described in Carl Senna's book, *The Fallacy of I.Q.*

During that five-year period children from poor, illiterate, low IQ parents, living in a markedly depressed area of the city, have shown a sustained high performance on a variety of tests administered from infancy through their fourth year. Their IQ's jumped by more than 50 percent with some of them achieving an IQ as high as 135.

Originally Dr. Heber and his team, including professionals from the fields of psychology, psychiatry, sociology, and speech therapy, set out to learn more about the link between mental retardation and poverty. Contrary to the commonly held belief that the high incidence of retardation was a reflection of the overall environment, Dr. Heber found the highest concentration

186

among mothers with low IQ. They also knew that children of mothers with IQ's under 80 not only tested out with a low IQ initially but continued to decline as they grew older. To anyone looking for a glib answer, the low IQ could easily have been blamed on heredity.

Dr. Heber and his team thought otherwise. The challenge was to start working with the children in infancy, within weeks of their return from the hospital with a comprehensive "intervention" program. Forty mothers, all with IQ's under 70, volunteered to participate. At first, teachers visited their homes daily directing most of their attention to the babies rather than the mother. Then, when the babies were three or four months old, both mothers and children began to participate in the program at the Infant Education Center.

Until his second birthday each child had his own teacher, and then he was placed in a class of five, then eight, and, by the fourth birthday, a class of eleven. The day was structured, the schedule well planned with enough flexibility to take care of the needs of each individual child. The curriculum included language, grammar, science, art, and music.

Meanwhile, the mothers continued to receive training not only in child care and homemaking, but in vocational skills as well. A few have since received jobs.

Careful testing of vocabulary, grammar, comprehension, motor skills, and IQ has been part of the program from the beginning. In every instance the children exposed to mental stimulation since infancy have shown a striking superiority to the control group, with IQ tests on an average *33 points higher* than the control group. Some tested as *high as 135.*

When Dr. Heber and his colleagues began their project they hoped they would be successful in preventing the intellectual decline to which most of these children would probably have been doomed. What they did not expect was that the four years of intensive education would produce a group of children that would learn faster than was normal for their age group.

187

Dr. Heber is cautious and modest about his accomplishments to date but excited about the implications. "We have seen a capacity for learning on the part of extremely young children," he says, "that previously would not have been believed possible."

The Milwaukee project is a dramatic example that prevention of a handicap, in this instance mental retardation, can be a reality.

The relative impact of environment versus heredity on IQ now begins to tip in favor of environment. The most searching and detailed analysis of this subject to date is the 1972 book *Inequality: A Reassessment of the Effect of Family and Schooling in America.* Harvard Professor Christopher Jencks and his co-authors conclude that about 45 percent of the variation in IQ in the United States population is due to variations in the genes, about 35 percent to variations in environment, and the remaining 20 percent on interaction between environment and genes. It is that 55 percent of a child's mental development that offers the basis for educational and social action.

The widespread claim that IQ remains stable throughout one's lifetime has been based on children tested when they first entered school. Is it inevitable that the growth registered by the Milwaukee children will come to a halt at the age of six? One answer is now coming from the University of California, Berkeley, Institute of Human Development, where the lives of several hundred persons have been followed for decades. One study started with sixty-one healthy babies before they left the hospital. They were subsequently examined and repeatedly interviewed in childhood, adolescence, and adulthood. At the age of thirty-six, of the original sixty-one, fifty-four were still in the study.

One of the most significant conclusions was that the *level of intelligence continued to rise at least until the age of thirty-six.* This was particularly true with the test which measured vocabulary and general information and the ability to comprehend—in other words, factors heavily dependent on the capacity to understand

and use words. They also found that superior play facilities, parental attitudes toward education, and harmony in the household were among the factors related to high IQ scores later in life.

While most of the men and women in the study have had a better than average socioeconomic background and scored above average in the mental tests, there were also in the group several whose childhood IQ's were in the 60's. They too continued to improve. One man never scored higher than the low 60's from the age of five to sixteen. After that his mental tests began to rise. At twenty-one he learned to read and by the time he was thirty-six he scored an overall IQ of 80 with a performance score of 92!

A large segment of the population never gets the advantages of the California children in the study and the under *100* IQ PhD's whose high school science teachers nurtured their dreams and hopes.

As far back as World War I, the armed forces recorded lower IQ scores for blacks than for whites. It was interesting, though, that blacks from some Northern states scored higher than whites from some Southern states. The problem of why and how IQ scores differ among various racial groups was revived again in the early 1960's, when a Florida State University psychologist tested 1,800 black children in five Southeastern states. Comparing their scores with the scores of white children from the same region, he found the black scores significantly lower. Other studies since also showed a difference, ranging from 10 to 20 points. Again the differences are smaller for Northern blacks.

Despite steadily growing evidence unmasking the limitations of IQ tests as pure objective instruments and denying the effect of environment, a belief emerged that blacks are genetically inferior.

In the winter of 1969, Professor Arthur Jensen, University of California, Berkeley, was the author of an article in the *Harvard Educational Review* on "How Much Can We Boost I.Q. and Scholastic Achievement?" He not only asked the question, but had the answer. Blacks score lower than whites on IQ tests (true); special programs of compensatory education have failed to close the gap (not true).

Were such ideas given serious consideration, the result could be a slowing down of, if not an abrupt halt to, educational programs that still have a long way to go before society can be sure that "the best has been tried and failed." Neither the quality nor the quantity of compensatory education has been as yet so great as to claim demonstrable results. While Jensen acknowledges that IQ tests are not culture-free, he argues that this is the way they should be since the children being tested will move into a culture bound by the standards measured by the tests. Jensen was later joined in his views by Harvard psychologist Richard Herrnstein.

Meanwhile, Dr. Shockley continues the efforts he initiated in 1966 to promote research that would prove the genetic inferiority of blacks. He has appealed to black leader Roy Wilkins for the cooperation of 100 to 200 "outstanding black intellectuals to permit blood samples to be taken for a scientific evaluation." What Dr. Shockley expects to find in the blood is not revealed.

Dr. Shockley has also repeatedly requested the National Academy of Sciences to look into the matter of IQ and race, but, as of November, 1973, and ad hoc committee interested in the genetics of behavior had not yet taken any action.

What purpose would such a study serve? None, in the opinion of many geneticists. Professors Walter F. Bodmer and Luigi Cavelli-Sforzia emphasize that the gap in environments will have to be substantially reduced first before the relationship of race to intelligence can be measured. ". . . no good case can be made for such studies on either scientific or practical grounds," they wrote in *Scientific American,* October, 1970.

Professor Jencks in his chapter "What Color is I.Q.—Intelligence and Race" in *The Fallacy of I.Q.* comments on the difference in IQ scores among other ethnic groups, with the observation that family outlook and training also contribute. "Jewish children . . . do better on I.Q. tests than Christians at the same socioeconomic level, but very few people conclude that Jews are genetically superior to Christians. Instead," he explains, "we conclude that Jews treat their children differently from Christians even when their occupations, incomes and education are the same."

Were you to apply some of the Jensen-Shockley thinking to your own family, it would mean that if one of your children has an IQ of 100 and another 115, you would accept the idea that the first child should have entirely different educational experiences, goals, occupation, and ultimate status in life from the second.

Perhaps the most pertinent question about IQ for each individual is "How much is my future success in life determined by my IQ?" The answer is: not as much as you have been led to believe. Indeed, *after* you have finished school, it will affect your success less than other factors. By that time (and admittedly IQ is a factor in determining what level of schooling you complete) other factors are far more important—the social class into which you are born, luck (you may work for a firm for twenty years which then goes out of business and even an IQ of 160 may not save you your job), the year you start your career (you would have had a brighter future in space science in 1964 than 1974). Not to be forgotten is your sex. An extra 15 points in IQ will not secure a job for a woman when a man is traditionally preferred.

It would not be at all surprising that the top industrialist in town, his chauffeur, his secretary and his doctor all have the same IQ. Other events in their lives have placed them where they are.

How much do you value a high IQ? Professor Jencks points out: "Low I.Q.'s are not the cause of American social problems and higher I.Q.'s would not solve these problems. Any white reader who doubts this should simply ask himself whether he would trade in his genes which make his skin white for genes which would raise his I.Q. 15 points."

Would you?

13

Schizophrenia
—A Distorted Reality

Josh was never what you would describe as a boisterous child, but neither was he so quiet and withdrawn as to attract your attention. He was a better than average student, whose teachers knew that even if he would make no spectacular contribution to the class, neither would he make trouble. Or so it seemed until his junior year at high school.

When the change came, it was not obvious at first. In contrast with an almost perfect attendance record for years, he began to miss more and more days of school. He was too tired to get up in the morning, because he had tossed most of the night neither asleep nor awake. He didn't complete homework assignments or start special projects.

The causes of the change were curious experiences which had begun rather suddenly and which he was not yet ready to tell his parents about. Only last Monday when he opened his school locker his key in the lock sounded so thunderously loud that he was thrown back as if he had been physically assaulted. As soon as he entered the audiovisual room where he worked in his free time, he knew at once that "they were all talking about him." As the days went on, he felt more and more isolated, as if he were waging a lonely war against enemies he could not identify. He could be threatened anywhere—at school, at the supermarket where he worked after school, in his own room at home.

By midyear he was failing virtually every course. He no longer trusted his ability to think rationally. Reluctantly he forced himself to accept the fact that the world he now inhabited was different from that of his family, friends, and schoolmates; it was a world in which he was helpless. He was later to describe his despair as "an endless and limitless nothingness."

When Josh's parents were asked to come to school to talk with the school psychologist, their reaction was mixed. To be sure, they had noticed his moodiness, his increasing apathy, and his long hours alone in his room. But, they assured each other, this comes with adolescence; it is a stage he is going through. On the other hand, they were concerned about the marked deterioration in his schoolwork and the constant fatigue to which they attributed it.

A visit to the family doctor ruled out the assurance they sought. "I hope I can help you, Josh," he said, "But I need help—yours, your family's, and a specialist who knows more about your condition than I do."

The condition is schizophrenia, a mental disorder that affects more than 2,000,000 Americans.

"It is predicted," writes Dr. Loren R. Mosher, chief of the Center for Studies of Schizophrenia, National Institute of Mental Health, "that 2% of persons born in 1960 will have an episode of schizophrenia sometime during their lives." And to that he adds the grim prediction that in slum areas the risk soars to 6 percent. Most vulnerable are young people between sixteen and thirty, but it also strikes very young children, as well as mature men and women.

194

While each of us perceives the world around us with a uniqueness that reflects our own interests, attitudes, and experiences, there is nevertheless a "reality" about which we generally agree. Not so for the schizophrenic whose perceptions at times of any or all of his senses—sight, sound, touch, taste, smell—are so distorted that his is a bizarre world bearing little resemblance to our reality.

His distorted perceptions shape the inappropriate behavior so common in this disorder. The queer taste of the food he is served triggers his fear of being poisoned. He hears voices that are not actually there, and they seem to constitute threats and plots against him.

Until not too long ago schizophrenia was regarded as an incurable disease. To the sense of hopelessness was added a sense of shame and guilt. "What did we do wrong?" has been the cry of countless parents like Josh's.

Very few psychiatrists today lay the major blame on parents' behavior for the development of schizophrenia. To be sure, severe strain in the family relationship usually develops by the time the patient reaches the doctor. Josh's mother's response ranged from an oversolicitous hovering to a quiet withdrawal and despair. His father was often remote and disapproving, as if to say, "I did my best—that's it."

Too much is known today about the biology and genetics of schizophrenia to describe it purely as a "breakdown in interpersonal relationships."

How much does heredity have to do with schizophrenia? The first serious attempt to apply genetics to this problem was launched at an international meeting of psychiatrists in 1917. The targets were schizophrenia (called dementia praecox at that time) and manic-depressive psychosis. Since then researchers have gathered much data confirming the genetic link. The disease occurs more commonly in both identical twins than in both fraternal twins and is also found more frequently among sisters, brothers, and cousins than in the general population. Moreover, schizophrenia is found with nearly the same degree of frequency in countries that are very different culturally and geographically, making it difficult to ascribe the illness to environmental conditions unique to one society.

Perhaps the most quoted and for many years unchallenged study was that by the noted geneticist Dr. Franz J. Kallman, who found in the 1940's that among identical twins, if one was schizophrenic, there was an 85 percent chance that the other would be also. Such a prophecy, of course, imposed a great fear in families with one affected twin. It was like waiting for the other shoe to drop.

More recent studies reveal that while heredity counts, its contribution is smaller than Dr. Kallman suggested. When researchers began to look at twins in the general population rather than among hospitalized patients, as Dr. Kallman did, the concordance (similarity in each twin of a pair) turned out to be considerably smaller.

Most revealing was a study of close to 16,000 pairs of twins who served in the armed forces of the United States during World War II and the Korean War. All were physically and mentally fit when inducted. A follow-up eighteen to twenty years later located more than 400 pairs in which schizophrenia had been diagnosed in either one or both members of the pair. Among identical twins the disorder had developed in both members in no more than 14 percent of the cases, while only among 4 percent of the pairs of nonidentical twins were both members affected. Thus it now appears that the probability for the other shoe dropping is markedly less than the 85 percent hitherto feared.

Until very recently the research on the causes of schizophrenia implicated both "nature" and "nurture" without yielding solid evidence to nail down how much each contributes. In addition to psychological and emotional trauma, scientists have identified risks imposed by complications of pregnancy and delivery, illness and accidents. Yet the basic question remains: Do children of schizophrenics become schizophrenic because they have been reared in a disturbed psychological setting or because of their own genetic makeup?

The first definitive answers are coming in from a ten-year collaborative study of adopted people in Denmark conducted by NIMH researchers Drs. David Rosenthal, Seymour Kety, and Paul Wender. When they looked into the backgrounds of thirty-three adult schizophrenics, all adopted early in life, they uncovered a significantly higher incidence of schizophrenia and other mental illnesses among their biologic relations than among their adopted relations. Mental illness was also more prevalent among their biologic relations than among biologic relations of adopted children who did not become schizophrenic.

Even more convincing evidence of the role of genes comes from a follow-up on children of schizophrenic parents adopted early in infancy and reared by nonschizophrenic adoptive parents. The percentage that developed schizophrenia (7 percent) was not too different from the percentage that became schizophrenic when reared by their own schizophrenic parents. Moreover, other mental aberrations afflicted an inordinately large number (23 percent) compared to a figure of only 10 percent so afflicted among adopted children whose biologic parents were not schizophrenic.

On the other hand, a point may also be scored for the benefits of "nurture." The researchers found evidence suggesting that despite the genetic handicap and its consequences, the vulnerable adoptees manage to function better in a normal environment than they would if left with a schizophrenic parent.

In their efforts to define the mode of inheritance, some geneticists have suggested a dominant gene with low penetrance. Others maintain it is a recessive gene, while a large number favor a group of genes, interacting with each other and with the environment. The definitive answer, however, remains elusive.

197

Sigmund Freud was among the first psychiatrists to maintain that schizophrenia is a disease with chemical abnormalities and that it would ultimately be treated successfully with the help of chemicals and drugs. His prophecy has been only partially fulfilled, although mounting evidence suggests that he was correct.

Evidence of faulty metabolism in the living brain is hard to come by. Much of the research in schizophrenia has been on other body tissues including blood, urine, muscle, and, most recently, spinal fluid. Among the more promising clues so far are the behavior of a group of chemicals (catecholamines) active in brain function and bearing a close similarity to hallucinogens; deficiency of an enzyme required for the normal breakdown of hallucinogens in the body; elevated blood levels of familiar muscle enzymes as well as changes in the muscle tissues of schizophrenics; reduced activity of an important nervous system enzyme (monoamine oxidase) in the blood platelets of schizophrenics.

The burgeoning use of mood-changing drugs in the 1960's provided psychiatrists with a new crop of man-made schizophrenic-like patients. LSD trips—both good and bad, with the perception changes enjoyed by some, and the horrifying hallucinations and distortions suffered by others—suggested to psychiatrists that they were dealing with a model of the disease. A closer look revealed more differences than similarities. When amphetamine abuse (especially speed, i.e., methamphetamine) became widespread, psychiatrists noted that amphetamine-induced psychoses were so close to the disease in nature that it was sometimes difficult to distinguish between the two.

While no single marker common to all schizophrenics (such as abnormal sugar metabolism in diabetics or abnormal milk metabolism in galactosemia) has been found to date, there is no longer any doubt about a biochemical basis for some of the bizarre behavior of the schizophrenic. And despite the lack of success in nailing down a specific cause for schizophrenia, dramatic strides have been made in its management. The first breakthrough came as a corollary of a routine observation of a new sedative designed to be used before surgery.

In 1951 a French anesthesiologist noted that surgical patients taking the new sedative were, although fully conscious, surprisingly free of anxiety and almost indifferent to the impending event. After surgery they were remarkably free of the usual postoperative restlessness. The new sedative was chlorpromazine—a synthetic drug that made its first appearance in 1950. It was not long before it moved from anesthesiology to psychiatry. Hyperactive, agitated, excited patients were calmed without clouding consciousness and without suffering impaired judgment.

One of the first to use it in the Western Hemisphere, Montreal's Dr. Heinz E. Lehmann, recalls that he could not believe his eyes. Not only did it calm, but in the acutely ill hallucinations and delusions were abolished.

The new tranquilizing drugs (chlorpromazine and others developed since) signaled a new era in the treatment of schizophrenia. For Josh it meant not a cure, but a dramatic change of mood that freed him from his emotional and mental prison. Not only could he begin to function better, but he could respond to psychotherapy more easily.

Like many other schizophrenics, he needed hospitalization before he could pick up his life at school and at home. In contrast with the premedication days, hospitalization is no longer a sentence that seems like a lifetime. Josh was admitted to a hospital close to home and during his six-week stay he received both individual and group therapy. At the same time his parents were asked to come in for sessions in family therapy (a technique receiving increasing acceptance) to help them learn to live better with their son's schizophrenia.

At about the same time that the new tranquilizers were introduced, another new treatment for schizophrenia was initiated by Drs. Abram Hoffer and Humphry F. Osmond of the University of

Saskatchewan. (Dr. Osmond is now the director of the Bureau of Research, New Jersey Neuro-Psychiatric Institute, Princeton.) Since 1952 they have been treating schizophrenics with large doses of Vitamin B_3, niacin. Since that time additional vitamins have been added.

By 1966 Drs. Hoffer and Osmond were able to report that a ten-year follow-up of 2,000 patients treated with vitamins revealed a 75 percent recovery rate compared to 36 percent without them. Reliance was not on megavitamins alone; the other remedies were not abandoned. Best results were obtained among patients whose illness was not of long duration and with those who had no family history of schizophrenia.

Although the large doses of vitamins used can do no harm and conventional treatment is continued, megavitamin therapy was and still is controversial. Many doctors refuse to use it, claiming that its efficacy has not yet been proved in a scientific manner. But a Long Island psychiatrist who adopted megavitamin therapy in 1966 initially for alcoholic schizophrenics and later for young people suffering the mental consequences of LSD, speed, and other drugs reports highly encouraging results. Dr. David Hawkins, medical director of the North Nassau Mental Health Center, Manhasset, New York, and director of psychiatric research at Brunswick Hospital Center, Amityville, has treated more than 4,000 schizophrenics at the clinic and more than 150 in the hospital, with an encouraging rate of success in both groups.

Megavitamin therapy is now also known as Orthomolecular Psychiatry—a term coined by Professor Linus Pauling, who believes that schizophrenics, despite a normal diet, may suffer from an inadequate supply of essential nutrients in the brain. This condition might be described as "cerebral deficiency disease," and he believes it is due to an inherited biochemical defect, like PKU and others. Massive doses of Vitamin B_3, B_6, C, and others can, in Dr. Pauling's opinion, correct the deficiency. While psychiatrists continue to debate the value of the vitamin treatment, many patients and their families continue to extol its virtues. The last word on it has clearly not been said.

Meanwhile, patients with schizophrenia continue to be the single largest group in mental hospitals, but the number of first admissions for the disease has decreased by more than 10 percent in recent years, in contrast with an increase of 36 percent in admissions for other mental disorders. However, for many schizophrenics discharge from the hospital continues to be through a revolving door. Because they are unable to make it back in the world, the readmission rate is very high.

Much is still to be learned. What is the nature of the genetic defect that predisposes to schizophrenia? What is the precise biochemical abnormality that accounts for the hallucination and the distorted perception? Is schizophrenia a single disease or, as it was first described in 1911, a "group of schizophrenias"? What determines that a boy like Josh develops schizophrenia and his brother and sister may not? What events in the home and the community help take the sting out of the illness, and what events make it worse?

Support for research in schizophrenia in this country has grown from $113,000 in 1948 to $10,000,000 in 1971. Is it enough?

Josh is one of the lucky ones for whom the combination of drug medication, individual psychotherapy, and family involvement is working. Today he is a sophomore in college and functioning satisfactorily. Cured? Like any other serious illness, the scars are there. He may have relapses, but if he does, he knows not only that the medication will help, but that there are people in the real world to whom he can turn when his own inner world becomes unreal again.

14

The Many Faces
of Mania and Melancholy

"I have two birthdays," says Mildred, "the date on my birth certificate and the date I was discharged from the psychiatric hospital three years ago." Her new birthday stems from a new treatment that promises her a future relatively free of the events that have made twelve years of her life a nightmare of recurrent attacks of melancholy and mania.

Mildred is a victim of manic-depressive psychosis—a group of mental disorders that, like schizophrenia, take many forms and faces. Today, more than half a century after psychiatrists began to look for the role that heredity plays (family studies convinced them that it was there), the pattern of transmission in some families is emerging. Moreover, it may now become possible to predict in these families who has inherited the vulnerability and who may escape it.

For Mildred the big news is lithium—an ancient remedy brought back to life after 1,500 years, a substance that has calmed her mania and, when taken as a daily dose, is successfully preventing depression.

Her first episode was only two weeks after she started college. Not quite seventeen, she seemed mature for her age. She had already shouldreed more responsibility than most teen-agers, taking care of her younger sister and brother as well as helping her mother in the family store during the periods her father was hospitalized for "nervous breakdowns." It was, in fact, a dream come true for her to have been permitted to go away to college.

One morning she hurriedly left her biology class, ran to the bank, and withdrew the $230 that were to see her through the next few months. She asked for the money in small bills. Her next destination was the main business street of the small college town, where she began to disburse the money at random. Pressing the money on bewildered passersby, she urged each one to take it, assuring them that there was much more where that came from.

The rest of the semester was spent at home, and the spring found her registered in a local commuting college. Her recovery however was short-lived. The next attack took the form of a deep depression. "I was worthless, a born loser," she recalls. "I felt like an exhausted swimmer going upstream against a strong current, knowing that I would never make it and not caring that I wouldn't."

Sometimes the two moods were uncomfortably close, switching in hours from weeks of silence, isolated from family and friends, to an excited, argumentative, hyperactive elation, when all things seemed possible—love, wealth, success.

For every victim like Mildred who suffers from both manic and depressed episodes, there are at least ten who suffer from depression alone.

Such a one is Arthur who, seven months after his father's death, was still mourning him with a sustained sorrow. He was not the only member of his family depressed by the sudden loss of the man they loved and admired. But by now his mother was back at her job at the local library, his sister was back at college, and even his grandfather to whom the loss of his only son was a crushing blow was working in the garden—"the plants need me."

Arthur alone was immobilized, indifferent to his wife-to-be, unmoved by the books and records he had enjoyed so much in the past, apathetic about his job. Indeed, just getting out of bed in the morning was a major task, and choosing a shirt and tie when he reluctantly dressed, a major decision. What had started as a normal, indeed a necessary, grief was now a severe depression. Arthur had shifted the focus of his sorrow from his father to himself.

There has been no history of mental illness in Arthur's immediate family, but it is known that a substantial number of all depressives have a blood relation with the same disease.

At least 125,000 Americans will be hospitalized for severe depression this year; more than 200,000 will receive treatment in doctors' offices and clinics. The numbers diagnosed and treated represent only the tip of the iceberg. Adding to the difficulty of reaching under the iceberg to melt it is the frequency with which depression is masked by physical complaints and the manner in which it is tangled up with alcoholism and with drug abuse.

Depression is a psychological backdrop for many of the 23,000 suicides in the United States each year.

What makes this dismal picture even sadder is that of all the mental disorders, depression stands out as the one that, once diagnosed, can be treated with a high degree of success.

In looking for the root causes of manic-depressive illnesses, scientists have turned up the same factors encountered in schizophrenia: environment, life experiences, stress, and a family history of the disease. In fact, repeated occurrences of depression within families, sometimes in three successive generations, implicates heredity even more strongly than in schizophrenia (90 percent of schizophrenics do not have a schizophrenic parent).

In recent years it has become popular to divide manic-depressives into two categories: those who, like Arthur, suffer only depression (unipolar), and those who, like Mildred, experience periods of both mania and depression (bipolar). Several investigators have suggested that when illness strikes a family, it will follow a pattern of either predominantly unipolar or predominantly bipolar. And so, if genes are involved, the implication is that there are at least two distinct genes. On the other hand, it has also been found that the lines are not always that clearly drawn, for both unipolar and bipolar manifestations have been found in the same family. As they have in Mildred's, whose aunt, her father's sister, went through several periods of severe depression before she developed cancer and died from it when not quite forty.

Even more puzzling are the identical twins with the illness where sometimes one twin is unipolar and the other bipolar. It may be that there is a single genetic predisposition, but that other factors come into play to determine the outcome.

Because so often the victim is a woman and because her sons and her daughters are more likely to be sick than the sons of an affected father, suspicion has focused on the existence of a dominant gene (only one is needed) on the X chromosome. From studies now in progress, a picture is beginning to emerge that speaks very strongly for just such a dominant gene.

Dr. Julien Mendlewicz and his colleagues at the New York State Psychiatric Institute studied the families of seven hospitalized manic-depressive patients. (Theirs was not the first such study, but it is the most thorough to date.) They interviewed spouses, parents, sisters and brothers, offspring, uncles, grandparents, cousins, and more distant relatives as well. In each family there had been mental illness in at least three generations. Each family incidentally had both unipolar and bipolar individuals.

What was even more striking was that some of the affected males were color-blind with a type of color blindness known to be transmitted by a gene on the X chromosome. The gene for color blindness is itself totally unrelated to the mental disorder but is located close enough to the gene for manic-depression to be transmitted with it (linkage).

It then becomes a marker. A few years ago it was reported that a particular blood group, X ga, is also on the X chromosome close to the gene for manic depression and that too serves as a marker.

One patient, also color-blind, has three brothers. Two are emotionally ill and color-blind. The oldest brother is neither ill nor color-blind. They recall that their mother was treated several times during her lifetime for depression. Their aunt, their mother's sister, suffered from bipolar depression and had in fact been hospitalized for mania. Two of her sons are neither depressed nor color-blind; the third is both.

If there is a dominant gene on the X chromosome, it explains why, when a woman herself is affected, there is a fifty-fifty chance in each pregnancy that she can transmit it to both her sons and daughters. An affected man who contributes his X chromosome to his daughters can also contribute the vulnerability to them. This may have been the story with Mildred and her father. There have been rare instances where both fathers and sons suffer from manic depression, and while there is as yet no explanation of the mode of transmission (only the Y chromosome goes to the son), the evidence for X transmission in other instances remains strong.

What this can mean to an affected family is underscored by an editorial in the *British Medical Journal,* April, 1973, pointing out if further studies reveal that a dominant sex-linked gene is one determinant of the manic-depressive condition, "there is an important practical consequence. In such families it becomes possible to predict with a fair probability which individuals are liable to be manic depressives and which not: boys who are not color blind have only a small risk, but others have a big risk." Does this new knowledge have a potential for genetic counseling? If yes, it is still too early to define it. It may, however, serve as an alert to the color-blind boy or man in such a family.

For as many years as man has recorded his behavior he has also recorded accounts of persons like Mildred and Arthur who exhibited the crippling effects of mania and melancholy. Among the earliest is the Biblical account of Saul, the first King of Israel, about 1000 B.C., whose mental disorder manifested itself not too long after he was chosen for that exalted position. Indeed, Saul's attention was first directed to David, a young Judean, when he was advised by his counselors to secure a skillful musician whose playing would "relieve his torments."

Centuries later the Greeks and Romans after them were still prescribing music and wine. Today, while psychotherapy and counseling continue to be crucial components of treatment, the use of drugs has added a new dimension—often the only key to successful psychotherapy.

Drugs in the treatment of depression came onto the scene about twenty years ago at about the same time as they dramatically changed the management of schizophrenia. And as in schizophrenia, some of the most important discoveries had elements of serendipity. Lithium for the manic-depressive made its debut a few years earlier, off to a faltering start but picking up an accelerated momentum in the 1970's.

In the early 1950's a new drug, isoniazid, was introduced for the treatment of tuberculosis. The response of the patients was remarkable. Not only was the infection halted, but the patients became quite exhilarated. Nurses and doctors were pleased and surprised to see them dancing in the halls. Researchers soon learned that the same drug that overcame the tuberculosis also acted as an antidepressant.

Isoniazid belongs to a group of compounds known as monoamine oxidase inhibitors. In the next few years another group of antidepressants were developed, different from the MAO inhibitors and in some ways and for some patients more suitable.

Nevertheless, there are still many whose depression is not relieved by drugs, psychotherapy, or both. When Arthur showed no signs of "snapping out of it" (spontaneous recovery can occur), he kept the appointment made for him with a psychiatrist. He did not have to be convinced he was sick; he only had to believe that he could be helped. He went through the gamut of antidepressive drugs and also ran the gamut of reactions—from A to Z—agitated to "zombie." Indeed, there were times when he seemed worse than ever.

It was only then that he allowed arrangements to be made for electroconvulsive shock therapy—ECT.

First introduced about thirty-five years ago, shock still evokes passionate reactions from both its advocates and detractors. Electrodes are placed at each side of the head, and a low voltage electric current is sent through the brain for a fraction of a second. With the old techniques the subsequent convulsions were sometimes strong enough to cause fractures. Today the technique has been so improved that the aspects that used to appall both patients and professional staff have been virtually eradicated.

In preparation for his treatment, Arthur was given a mild anesthetic and a muscle relaxant. With milder convulsions, the danger of fractures is nil. He awoke after the treatment relaxed and rested but somewhat troubled by a slight loss of memory. This, he was soon to learn, is a frequent side effect but transient. "I could see the old Arthur beginning to emerge," his sister remarked.

Even very severe depressions respond dramatically in four to eight treatments. Arthur required the minimum.

How it works is still not understood. In the opinion of many of the detractors, tampering with the brain in an unexplained manner remains unacceptable. Perhaps the staunchest supporters are the patients themselves. For Arthur, shock meant the difference between a vegetative, nonproductive existence and return to a job and life with the involvement and capability that had been his before the depression overwhelmed him.

During the years of Mildred's bouts with depression, she too received shock. The benefits for her were minimal. She had been sick for ten years before lithium carbonate—an old drug with a new use—became available to her. This was the event that made possible what Mildred calls her new birthday.

Almost 1,500 years ago manic patients were sent to drink alkaline spring waters that must have been high in lithium. The tradition persisted for a few centuries and then faded into obscurity. Its ressurection in modern times was by an Australian psychiatrist, Dr. John F. J. Cade, in the late 1940's.

His early results with one patient were so encouraging that he tried it with others, and before the year was over he was able to note dramatic improvement in all ten. The lithium appeared to affect them all the same way: The mania subsided in those on the drug, but when the drug was withdrawn, the mania returned. Most striking was the observation that while the extreme hyperexcitability was successfully curbed, the patients were not sedated in the usual sense of the word. They were normally alert and responsive.

Dr. Cade's successes were soon duplicated by psychiatrists in Australia, France, Italy, and Denmark. In the United States, however, researchers did not rush to explore the possibilities of lithium, probably because it had earned a bad reputation in this country for reasons totally unrelated to mental illness. In the late 1940's lithium found its way to the tables of many Americans with heart disease and high blood pressure. Warned by their doctors to cut down on their salt (sodium chloride) intake, they found lithium chloride a tasty, inexpensive, and easily available substitute.

Lithium can easily be toxic in high doses, and patients receiving it therapeutically are monitored regularly with blood tests for lithium content. Some who used it at that time as a seasoning were not aware of the danger and exceeded the safe limit with regrettable consequences. The medical literature reported a number of poisonings, and three deaths were attributed to it. The

210

public was warned about the hazard, and lithium chloride was withdrawn from the market.

And so at just about the time that Dr. Cade and psychiatrists in various parts of the world were reporting success with the first specific chemical treatment for mental disease (it predated the phenothiazines soon to be so helpful with schizophrenics and the antidepressants as well) in the United States, lithium was in disrepute. Later, when investigators looked more closely into the poisonings and deaths associated with it in the United States, they learned that exceedingly large quantities far beyond the average accounted for some of the mishaps. The fright generated was so widespread that some of the symptoms attributed to lithium were in fact due to other causes.

Meanwhile, evidence of what lithium was accomplishing for manic-depressives in Europe and Australia continued to mount. Within a few days after treatment started, chaotic mood and behavior gave way to self-control, with rational thought restored. In contrast with three to four hours of restless, shallow sleep, patients were now able to sleep seven to eight hours a night; nor did they look or act drugged under its influence. Among those who benefited were some whose illness was recent, others with illness of long standing, including a sixty-one-year-old woman who had been hospitalized for thirty-five years. Lithium could no longer remain outside the pale of respectable drugs in the United States. By 1965 it received its first trial at the University of Texas and is now being used all over the country. Reports from ongoing studies point to a bright future for its use.

Today encouraging results continue to come in from the studies with the drug. A March, 1973, report in the *Archives of General Psychiatry* tells of 205 patients, most of whom had suffered previous episodes of mania, depression, or both. At the start of the program all were hospitalized with a manic episode. While in the hospital they all were stabilized on maintenance doses of lithium and then discharged. Then half the patients were continued on the lithium, and the other half were given a placebo (an innocuous substance). They all came back periodically for checkups and monitoring. The difference between the two groups was unmistakable. Lithium was twice as effective as the placebo in preventing relapse.

By the end of the second year 73 percent of the patients on lithium experienced *no* relapse in contrast with only 35 percent on the placebo.

Among psychiatrists who are still skeptical about lithium, even hostile (as was Mildred's therapist before her hospitalization when the lithium was first administered), an increasing number are coming around to the point of view that "it is worth trying, certainly for patients who might have had no other chance at a normal life."

In the last decade, the use of the drug to prevent recurrent attacks of mania and melancholy has been adopted in a number of countries. In Denmark between 1,000 and 2,000 patients receive a daily dose of lithium and report in faithfully for periodic checkups to make sure the dose is both effective and safe. They are, like Mildred, leading normal lives.

Lithium is not a cure all for all manic-depressives. At New York State Psychiatric Institute, one of the earliest to try it in the United States, early reaction was guarded. By 1972 in his *Journal of the American Medical Association* family study, Dr. Mendlewicz was able to describe the patient most likely to benefit: one who is still young when the first attack strikes, has a family history of the disease, and runs a more severe course of the illness.

Mildred fits into that category. She is doing well enough so that in the last three years since her treatment began she has been able to establish a successful business as a designer of needlepoint. She also plans to be married soon. No longer living with her family, she feels secure enough to put down her own family roots now. Does her future include children? For the present, she is leaving the options open.

Mildred and Arthur may confront stressful events in their future that are beyond their control. What they can do to help themselves is to know their own strengths and weaknesses—and recognize that their illness is not completely due to the genes, their biology, and their behavior. The outside world can both harm and help.

Some small starting steps have already been taken to help. There is a slowly growing understanding of both the anguish and treatability of mental illness. Public figures who are victims have been candid in talking of their experiences.

Some are functioning in high government places; others continue to be creative in the arts. Science too has a long way to go, but by now it has its direction—the chemistry, pharmacology, neurophysiology, and psychology of mental illness. A new professional organization, The Society to Conquer Mental Illness, made its debut in the spring of 1974 at a seminar with the theme "A Biological View of Mental Illness." Areas of concern include the genetics, biochemistry, and neurophysiology of mental disorders.

Millions of men, women, and children need their answers now.

15

XYY—One Male Chromosome Too Many

Scientists knew enough about chromosomes in 1961 to realize that an individual with fewer or more than the normal forty-six was in trouble. They were familiar with the mental retardation and other handicaps in Down's syndrome (forty-seven), the menstrual problems, infertility, and short stature of the Turner's syndrome (forty-five) female with only one X chromosome; the "superfemale" XXX (forty-seven), often with mental deficits and fertility problems as well; and the long-legged XXY male (Klinefelter's syndrome, (forty-seven)—usually with normal intelligence and sexual function but frequently infertile.

Not so with the first man in history with forty-seven chromosomes to be identified as an XYY. Despite the extra Y male-determining chromosome in every one of his cells, he had no discernible physical or psychiatric problems. He was a tall man of average intelligence, with a tendency to obesity, whose biggest problem seemed to be difficulty in keeping a job. He had been tested only because of an inordinate number of physical and mental abnormalities among his seven living offspring from two marriages. Scientists were still puzzled when a second normal XYY man was described later that year.

Four years were to pass before the XYY chromosome was to be associated by scientists with a disposition to aggression, violence, and crime. In 1965 Dr. Patricia Jacobs and her colleagues identified 7 XYY's among 197 mentally retarded men with criminal records confined to a maximum security hospital in Scotland. Two more were subsequently identified in the same institution. Six of the 9 were over six feet tall, 8 of the 9 of low intelligence, and most had exhibited aggressive or violent behavior on frequent occasions in the past. All had personalities characterized by extreme irresponsibility and instability, incapable of tolerating even the mildest frustration.

Dr. Jacobs' startling observations set off a search for XYY men in penal and psychiatric institutions elsewhere. In the next few years dozens of studies in Europe, the United States, and Australia confirmed that the proportion of XYY men behind bars in penal-psychiatric institutions *is* significantly higher than the 1 in 1,000 XYY found in the general population.

The public began to read about the new syndrome—the tall man with the extra male chromosome, often scarred with acne, prone to violence, crime, and aggression. Scientists, meanwhile, were beginning to get a somewhat different picture of the XYY man in trouble, but before there was an opportunity to put the mass of new observations into perspective, the issue took on a new sensationalism when it was implicated in three widely reported crimes.

Early in 1968 a Frenchman on trial for murder in Paris claimed that he was not criminally responsible for his behavior because he was an XYY. His trial ended with a verdict of guilty, but the judge was presumably persuaded that the extra Y chromosome bore some of the guilt, and the convicted man received a reduced sentence.

216

Not too long after that an XYY man was tried for murder in Melbourne, Australia. He was acquitted of murder for reason of insanity. Although it was reported in the press that his chromosomal abnormality was a key factor in the trial, his attorney only mentioned it in passing. His XYY played only a minor role in his defense, for there was ample medical evidence for insanity.

The most sensational story came from Chicago in the fall of 1968. An intruder into an apartment occupied by eight young nurses brutally murdered each one during a long terror-filled night. Even before he went on trial, there were stories that Richard Speck was an XYY and that it would be the basis for his defense. He fit the physical description of the XYY's identified in institutions—a tall man with acne. He went to trial, was convicted for murder, and sentenced to the maximum allowed by law.

While XYY played a major role in newspaper accounts about Richard Speck, the story behind the headlines is that it never came up in his trial. If he was tested, there is no record of it. The myth, however, did not die easily. Four years later, *Medical Tribune* published a letter from the chief of the laboratory of the Chicago hospital where the test is supposed to have been performed, denying that any such test had been performed on Speck.

Meanwhile, the XYY male was shaping up as a new threat to a society already gripped by fear of rising crime. A law journal of one of the nation's leading law schools even discussed the possible "preventive detention of all XYY's."

In the light of today's knowledge, how realistic are these fears? The final answer may not be determined for decades.

"The association of criminality and XYY is not true," asserts Dr. Digamber S. Borgaonkar, head of the Chromosome Laboratory and an associate professor at Johns Hopkins University School of Medicine, whose work is shedding new light on what it means to be an XYY. The picture that emerges now of the XYY is a man or a boy who, while he may be taller than his parents or brothers, is not noted for his excessive tallness; is probably white, from middle- or lower-middle-class background; is not necessarily mentally deficient (one has an IQ of 125, and almost half of those studied have IQ's over 100; is not necessarily aggressive (some are quite peaceful). But, all exhibit the personality characteristics Dr. Jacobs described in her original report—a man or boy who cannot stand stress, is extremely impulsive, whose control of his behavior, particularly when triggered or trapped, is markedly diminished.*

It is often the hard-to-control impulse that leads to the antisocial act. Caught and convicted, the XYY becomes another statistic.

Emphasizing the increased vulnerability of the XYY, Dr. Borgaonkar warns that "within the same family the XYY has a larger risk of breaking down than his XY brother."

Dr. Borgaonkar's experience with XYY's who have already manifested psychiatric or antisocial behavior (including sexual offenses) convince him that "knowing about XYY helps both the patient and his family to cope." In some instances the families' feeling of guilt that they had done something wrong was removed when they learned of the abnormality.

Only one family decided to deny the existence of the abnormality and its possible implication for their son's behavior. Dr. Borgaonkar reassured the boy himself and told him he could "come back when you feel that trouble is ahead. We shall be here to help you."

With so much still unknown about the XYY it is not surprising that there is a difference of opinion among doctors about how it should be handled. "Discovery of an extra Y sex chromosome in a male hardly predicts anti-social behavior with the confidence . . . that the trisomy 21 [mongolism] predicts mental retardation," writes Dr. Ernest B. Hook, New York State Birth Defects Insti-

* A composite picture drawn by a Johns Hopkins team of thirty-five XYY's in prison reveals a broken family; school history of behavior problems; average IQ; excessive daydreamer; socially a loner; occupationally a drifter with unrealistic future expectations; impulsive in sexual expression, but lacking in depth of affection. Too few nonwhites have been identified to provide a composite picture of them.

tute, in *Science,* January, 1973. Sometimes, in his opinion, the knowledge can induce more difficulties and problems.

The doctor's dilemma is even greater when he learns from an amniocentesis that his pregnant patient is carrying a boy with XYY. *Medical World News* asked its physician readers if they would tell if they had such information and what they thought the consequences would be. Of the 150 doctors who answered, 139 said they would tell. Only 11 would keep the information to themselves.

For at least one doctor it was not a hypothetical situation, Dr. Hook reports. During the course of amniocentesis for the possibility of Down's syndrome, a prominent Chicago geneticist found that the fetus was an XYY. The mother was told what little was known of the prognosis, but it was enough for her. Her decision was to abort.

What are the factors that determine whether the 1 in 1,000 baby born with XYY will eventually manifest deviant behavior or melt into the ranks of the tens of thousands who never come to anyone's attention because nothing in their lives sets them apart?

Some scientists are now in the midst of a "prospective" study: find the XYY in infancy and watch him as he grows. How does he develop? Does he become antisocial and, if so, at what age? What has happened to him in his family, school, and experiences? At least seventeen male children are being followed from birth. Some are now six or seven years old, and the next few years may be crucial in the light of published accounts of deviant behavior in XYY boys of nine or ten.

In an effort to overcome the time lag imposed by studying the newborn or the very young, Dr. Borgaonkar has begun to look into a large school population in almost a dozen elementary schools, three junior high schools, and one senior high school in the city of Baltimore. The integrated school population consists of students from diversified economic backgrounds.

When Dr. Borgaonkar finds an XYY among the schoolchildren, he makes an appointment for a personal candid discussion with the parents. To the parent who asks, "What does it mean if my boy is an XYY?" he answers that under conditions of stress the extra Y chromosome may be a contributing factor to disturbed behavior. This knowledge could well be the first step in prevention.

At the present time the one aspect of the XYY that scientists agree upon is the extreme variability with which it expresses itself. Among them are some who are completely normal, others severely disturbed; some are tall, others average; some have acne, others clear skins; some are violent, others quiet. Some produce an excessive amount of male sex hormone, others a normal amount, and still others a decreased amount.

For the reader who may worry that there are thousands of dangerous men and boys walking the streets who should be locked up Dr. Borgaonkar's answer is "not just for being an XYY. After all, we accept a great deal of variability in the XY, why not in the XYY?"

16

Huntington's Disease

Once described by a critic as a "national possession like Yellowstone and Yosemite," folk singer Woody Guthrie left a legacy of more than 1,000 songs when he died in the fall of 1967. Woody will be remembered, however, by more than his songs, for his death lifted from obscurity one of the most disabling and destructive of all genetic diseases—Huntington's chorea (now also known as Huntington's disease—HD).

From the moment Woody's illness was correctly diagnosed, Marjorie Guthrie lived not only with the certainty of his death, but also with the knowledge of the risk to their three young children. Arlo, Joady, and Nora each have a 50–50 chance of having inherited the defective gene responsible for the disease. And if they have, it can be as long as fifteen to twenty years before they find out.

HD is a fatal degenerative neurological disorder that strikes both men and women. It can be inherited from either father or

221

mother and can be transmitted to both sons and daughters. Only a single dose is required (dominant) for it to show up. There is no generation gap; whoever inherits the gene inherits the disease. Unlike other genetic disorders like PKU, galactosemia, etc., that make their presence known shortly after birth, it may be thirty-five to forty years before HD manifests itself. By then the sufferer may already have passed the defective gene on to his children, who may in turn be trapped in the relentless chain. One New England family has produced eleven successive generations with chorea.

The nature of the disease and the pattern of transmission within families was first described with rare insight by twenty-two-year-old Dr. George Huntington in 1872. Both his father and grandfather were physicians, and he was still a boy when he first saw an affected mother and daughter in East Hampton, Long Island. "Hereditary chorea," he wrote, "is confined to certain and fortunately few families, an heirloom from generations away back in the distant past. . . . It is spoken of by those in whose brain the seeds of the disease are known to exist, with a kind of horror."

The disease was brought to America in the seventeenth century by English immigrants who settled in and around Boston. Almost 1,000 affected individuals from the New England area have traced their ancestry to four families. Some of the women among them were tried and hanged as witches in the Salem trials, so frightening was their erratic behavior to the Establishment. The daughter of one of the original settlers moved down to East Hampton, and probably Dr. Huntington's patient was one of her descendants.

The first sign of the disease may be a change in personality—irritability, moodiness, and oversensitivity to slights both real and imagined. Then come involuntary movements of the face, hands, and shoulders; initially within the limits of just "fidgeting," they deteriorate to wild and uncontrolled flailing (hence the name chorea from the Greek word for "dance"). Facial expressions become grotesque.

222

As the disease progresses, speech thickens and becomes unintelligible. The victim loses the ability to control his muscles and eventually becomes totally disabled. As a final blow, most of those afflicted, but not all, suffer complete mental deterioration. The destruction of the part of the brain that controls muscles has now spread to the part of the brain that controls rational thinking. Woody was among those who was sane until he died, but toward the end he could barely respond. When Marjorie told him that Arlo was to give his first rock concert at Carnegie Hall, only the blink of an eye communicated his pleasure.

One of the most tragic aspects of the disease is that it kills slowly. For Woody it took thirteen years.

When word got out that Woody was a patient at New York's Creedmoor State Hospital, a victim of the disease, letters began to pour in. Most were from families to whom the disease was no stranger—as it was to many doctors and the general public. They wrote of their isolation, their fears, and their despair. Nothing was known about what caused it, how to prevent it, how to treat it. No hope could be held out for the victim, no guidance for the threatened family.

Woody was already almost completely incapacitated when Marjorie met for the first time with a group of affected families, physicians, and representatives from medical agencies. From that meeting grew the Committee to Combat Huntington's Disease (CCHD)—an event that was to be the turning point for thousands of victims and their families. By bringing out into the open what has long been a hush-hush condition, the committee is helping them deal with their crushing burdens in a realistic way. For the first time in history, sons, daughters, wives, grandchildren, and the patients themselves know that they are not alone.

What does a mother tell her son who has just called with the good news that his wife is pregnant when only yesterday she has learned that her husband's long-standing illness has finally been diagnosed as HD? Now both her son and his unborn baby are potential victims. How does a father tell his two daughters engaged to be married that their mother has HD? Can it be explained to their prospective husbands? Can they contemplate parenthood with the specter of their own vulnerability, as well as that of their future children? What do you tell a six-year-old who laughs at his father's sloppiness at the table and clumsiness in moving about the house? What can you tell the nineteen-year-old college sophomore who learned to love athletics from the father who is now no longer able to walk, much less race around a tennis court?

Today they are getting some of the answers from the network of forty-one CCHD chapters across the country and from the sharpened awareness among doctors about HD. In the first five years of CCHD more research was inspired and supported than in the ninety-five years since the disease was first described.

Joseph knew exactly what the future held when the neurologist confirmed what he had suspected for some time—HD. His father's bizarre behavior and final deterioration before his death were still fresh memories. Now he had to confront a whole new set of problems. How much longer could he be the breadwinner? The boys were twelve and fourteen, the girl only eight. How would his wife cope with her new role in the family? Despite some ominous signs in the months preceding the diagnosis, they avoided any mention of the disease. The doctor's verdict, however, changed all that. Even before they reached home, they had already begun to talk and plan for the future.

Today, four years later, Joseph continues to maintain a far higher level of activity and independence than he had initially hoped for. With the help of palliative drugs, some of the abnormal body movements are diminished. A program of exercise helps keep him fit. His pride in his wife and children is his best tonic by far.

She has completed her master's in social work and is now on the staff of the local hospital. All the children know how serious their father's illness is—each on his own level. Only the oldest knows now of its hereditary nature. The younger boy realizes that while his father will never be able to take the bike trip they used to talk about or toss a ball around with him, they can still enjoy pro football on TV together. He is never too busy to provide an audience for the plays his daughter turns out at an astonishing rate. No matter what the future holds, both Joseph and his wife are determined that the children will know the whole picture without evasion, without distortions. They will have to be prepared to ask their own questions and make their own decisions.

If these children were ready for genetic counseling today, they would soon learn that the tools and techniques proved so successful in other disorders cannot be applied to HD. A recurrent plea from many doctors and patients alike has been: "If we only had a test to tell us in advance who can safely have children and who cannot. . . ."

In June, 1972, an international team of neurologists disclosed in the *New England Journal of Medicine* that they had a test that promised to detect the defective gene years before the symptoms appear. Twenty-eight men and women, the youngest seventeen and the oldest thirty-three, all with an affected parent, asked to be tested. Included in the study were twenty-four unaffected volunteers, among them husbands and wives of those at risk.

When small doses of L-dopa (the Parkinson syndrome medication) were administered, about one-third of the "testees" developed chorea-like movements. When the medication was withdrawn, the chorea disappeared. The volunteer controls had no reaction at all to the L-dopa. The transient chorea, the researchers believe, is the clue to the defective gene.

If the test is valid, it should now be possible to say to the eighteen who had no reaction, "You are safe, there is no HD in your future or that of your children." But what of the other ten? For them it is now a death watch until symptoms develop.

How do threatened young people feel about taking such a test? Says a young medical student who has just learned that his father has HD, "*No.* Right now I feel I can enjoy and hope for the normal fifty percent. If I were to learn that I was definitely going to get the disease, I believe that the rest of the normal years would be destroyed by it. At least by not knowing, I have a fifty percent chance of living a normal life and can be happy clinging to that fifty percent."

It became clear that the procedure is not merely a test for genetic counseling but a diagnostic procedure that says to a healthy and worried young person, "You are doomed to develop a fatal illness in ten or twelve years. Meanwhile, there is nothing we can do for you while you are waiting."

The researchers decided to suspend the tests until concrete help is available for the potential victim.

The dilemma of the genetic counselor working with the day-to-day problems of patients and their families is often deeper and not so easily solved.

Since the emergence of genetic counseling as a medical specialty, the recurrent theme of the counselor has been to assemble the best available information, impart it with compassion and clarity, and then stand back and allow the affected family to make the decision that they feel is best for them. After twenty years of counseling HD families, a nationally renowned authority on the disorder, Dr. John S. Pearson, Wichita, Kansas, is now taking a searching look into the consequences of the "laissez-faire" approach.

Deeply troubled by the large number who continue to rear families despite the knowledge that they themselves may develop the disease and the risk of transmitting it to their children, Dr. Pearson asks, "Why?" The counselor himself often contributes to these decisions by his efforts to blunt the horror of the presence of the HD gene. (Understandable considering the high suicide rate in HD.) The counselor finds himself giving such reassurances as: "You have just as good a chance of escaping the disease as of having it; thirty to forty years of a normal life can make whatever comes later acceptable; science will find an answer."

To be sure, there is hope that science *will* find an answer, but it has not so far. Many *do* develop the disease and come to question whether the thirty good years are not too large a price to pay for the fifteen of inevitable deterioration accompanying the bad.

These reassurances, Dr. Pearson contends, serve only as the "foundation for a decision to live it up and have children as if the risk of HD had never existed."

He now takes a clear and unequivocal stand against reproduction by members of HD families. In the past when asked, "What would you do in my place?" he, like many other counselors, avoided a direct answer. Today he answers without hesitation that in the same shoes he would by all means avoid having children. If that information is received with any degree of warmth, he quickly makes it clear that he will help in adoption, sterilization, or whatever further action is required to help implement the decision of no more births.

Experience with two generations of HD families convinces Dr. Pearson that individuals at risk who have made the decision early in life not to have their own children made a happier adjustment in the years ahead, even when time proved that they did *not* have the defective gene and that their own children would have been in no danger. Acknowledging that the final decision still remains with the people seeking guidance, Dr. Pearson nevertheless maintains that it is also the duty of the counselor to pass on his experiences about the greater happiness achieved by those who took *no* chances.

What are the prospects for the future for the family with HD? A participant at the 1972 World Federation of Neurology noted that "we meet today in an atmosphere of optimism which has never before occurred in HD." The scientists' optimism stems partially from the accelerated rate of research in HD and partially from the progress scored in related neurologic and genetic disorders in recent years.

The optimism is reflected in the day-to-day lives of thousands of families from whom the centuries-old stigma is gradually being erased. They get new reassurances from better-informed doctors, from an increased awareness of nurses and therapists, and from sharing experiences with other affected families.

Arlo Guthrie continues to reach millions not only with his music but with his message about HD. Nora is carving a successful career following in her mother's footsteps as a dancer. (Marjorie is a Martha Graham-trained professional.) Joady too has inherited the sensitivity and creativity of both of his parents. All three have also inherited the inner strength that kept Woody going in his last agonizing years and that has sent Marjorie out on the road with unflagging faith against a formidable foe—HD.

In one of Woody's beloved songs, "Why Oh Why?" a child asks, "Why don't you answer my questions?" "Because I don't know the answer" is the adult's frustrated response. A look into the future promises that the day may not be far off when HD will join the growing number of genetic disorders with their long-sought-after answers for survival.

17

The Future
—Promises and Problems

If Mendel, Miescher, and Garrod (Chapter 1) were on the scene today, they would be astonished at the consequences of their early discoveries in genetics: the revelation of DNA, the basic material of heredity; how DNA controls the orderly processes of life; the leap from Dr. Garrod's 4 inborn errors to 2,000 genetic disorders now identified.

Indeed, so rapid is the accumulation of new knowledge that scientists are talking about procedures that were not in the vocabulary only a decade ago: gene therapy, enzyme replacement, cellular engineering, etc.

For the most part, managing genetic diseases today relies on changing the immediate environment in which the faulty gene functions. When a galactosemic cannot handle milk, remove milk and milk products from his diet; if a thalassemic cannot manufacture enough healthy red blood cells, make up the deficit with blood transfusions; when a hemophiliac bleeds for lack of a clotting factor, replace it. In each instance the defective gene is still there and functioning; the palliative measure only thwarts its harmful consequences.

Now, however, the first steps have been taken to go beyond palliation and toward correcting the basic errors. Scientists are no longer asking if it can be done but, rather, when.

The prospect of correcting the garbled information in a defective gene has excited geneticists since the 1950's, when Dr. Joshua Lederberg (now a Stanford University Nobel Laureate) discovered that a virus can carry a piece of genetic information from one bacterium to another (transduction). Every time you are infected with a virus it injects itself into one of your cells and substitutes its genetic information for your own. A disease-causing virus may kill the cell it infects, and the viral information is no longer a part of you. Sometimes, however, the virus is only a harmless "passenger" moving from one cell to another. Its genetic information becomes entrenched and is now a permanent part of the genetic information of the cell it inhabits. Would it be possible, Dr. Lederberg speculated, for a harmless virus with correct genetic information for a particular enzyme to take the place of the incorrect instructions in the defective gene?

Two conditions had to be met to try out the theory: a harmless virus with a message for an enzyme, and somebody with a genetic disorder attributed to a deficiency of that enzyme. The first condition was met many years ago with the discovery of a virus that causes warts in rabbits (Shope papilloma virus) and makes large quantities of the enzyme arginase. The researchers knew it was harmless to man because the laboratory workers infected with it either accidentally or deliberately suffered no ill effects. Once in the body, the enzyme went to work and broke down the amino acid arginine, also an innocuous effect. The viral message appeared to be incorporated for decades.

Many years were to pass before the second condition for gene therapy was to be met: a disease attributed to the missing or defective enzyme. In 1969 just such a situation came to Dr. Lederberg's attention. A German pediatrician was taking care of two sisters, one five years old and the other eighteen months. Both were severely mentally retarded with many physical complications. Both had exceedingly high levels of the amino acid arginine in their blood, suggesting a deficiency of the enzyme arginase. Possibly the search for a use for the enzyme in the Shope virus was over. And if it worked, the children could still be helped.

Dr. Lederberg lost no time in contacting the veteran researcher in Shope papilloma virus, Dr. Stanfield Rogers. He told him about the children in Germany with the first reported condition of too much arginine. The rest was up to Dr. Rogers in Oak Ridge, Tennessee, and Dr. H. G. Terhaggen in Cologne, Germany.

When they injected the virus into the sisters in 1970 and again the following year, their blood level of arginine was brought down. *The message to make the enzyme arginase seemed to have gotten through.* Unfortunately, the mental and physical improvement did not parallel the biochemical improvement. Perhaps the correction came too late. Meanwhile, despite advice about the continuing risk of its happening again, the couple had another child in 1971—again a little girl with the enzyme deficiency. She too received the Shope virus, but her progress is not encouraging. Perhaps the damage is already irreversible while the baby is still in utero.

The reaction to the use of the virus to cure a defect in a gene aroused a flurry of excitement among scientists. Some applauded the effort despite the disappointing clinical benefits. Others questioned the wisdom of introducing a virus whose safety by injection to humans over a long period of time has not yet been established.

In a 1972 interview with Dr. Rogers he defended the use of the virus in this particular family. "It is not too different from the live virus we use in vaccinations all the time, except that our preparation is purer. Moreover," he continued, "we always measure benefit against risk in medicine, and these little girls were doomed without it." As for the safety of the Shope virus, Dr. Rogers pointed out: "I was infected in '35, still had a low blood arginine in '55, and the level did not come back to normal until '65." He continues to show no ill effects to this day.

Another attempt at gene therapy is in progress in the research laboratories of the National Institute of Mental Health. In 1971 Dr. Carl Merril and his associates reported an initial success in introducing a correct genetic message into cells from a galactosemic patient (see Chapter 11).*

Dr. Merril cultured the human galactosemic cells in the laboratory and then exposed them to a virus that had picked up a correct message for the missing enzyme from a bacterium it had previously infected. The new generations of human galactosemic cells originally unable to make the enzyme began to produce detectable amounts. By the fall of 1973 Dr. Merril reported at the Fourth International Conference on Birth Defects in Vienna that he had achieved the same success with cells from other galactosemics.

Dr. Merril's work has not yet been confirmed by other scientists who tried to duplicate it, but if it stands up, it will be the first "cure" of a defective gene in a test tube, to be translated, it is hoped, in time to medical use as well.

An entirely different approach to gene therapy comes from Columbia University's Dr. Paul Marks, whose goal is to correct genetic defects in hemoglobin production (Chapter 4, sickle cell disease, and Chapter 8 thalassemia). Unlike Dr. Rogers and Dr. Merril, who depend on a virus to carry the message, Dr. Marks uses a sample of purified messenger RNA to carry the proper instructions back into the DNA in the nucleus of the cell. So far

---

* Because of the inheritance of a double dose of a defective gene needed to produce an enzyme used to break down milk and milk products, the galactosemic suffers mental retardation, cataracts, and sometimes early death.

232

there is encouraging evidence of new DNA with the correct information. The next step will be to find out if the repaired DNA will send out its new message. If it works, it will mean new hope for millions with the defective genes of SS disease and thalassemia.

Also in the future of gene therapy is a development based on the chance discovery in the 1960's that two different cell lines cultured in the laboratory could fuse and grow together—hybrids. Experiments are now going on to fuse the cells of patients with defective genes with cells from normal individuals, in the hope that the hybrid will develop the normal enzyme. Returning the cells to the patient may then provide him with the correct gene.

Cell hybridization is already yielding rich rewards in basic research. While the original hybrids were from two parent lines of the same species, scientists can now grow hybrids of man and mouse, man and hamster, and others.

In contrast with gene therapy which is still in the experimental stage, the technique of cellular engineering in genetic disorders, introduced only a few years ago, continues to save lives. David was the thirteenth male child born in his mother's family with a genetic defect that stripped him of his defenses against infection (combined immunodeficiency disease). Like the twelve preceding him, his prospects of surviving infancy appeared dim. Today, however, David is an active healthy six-year-old whose genetic defect has been overcome to the extent that he has his own functioning system of immunity, and to whom a cold is a sniffle, not a life-threatening event of major proportions.

When he was five months old, David contracted pneumonia and, despite massive doses of antibiotics, showed no hope of rallying. In desperation his parents flew him to Minnesota to the one man who probably knew more about David's condition than anyone in the country—pediatrician and immunologist Dr. Robert A. Good (now director of the Sloan Kettering Institute for Cancer Research). Dr. Good recognized that there was only one

233

chance for David—a transplant of healthy bone marrow cells that would, he hoped, replace the defective cells in his marrow responsible for his lack of immunity.

Without a perfectly matched donor the procedure itself could be a hazard to the sick baby. There was no perfect donor, but one of David's three older sisters, Doreen, was close enough to take a chance on. Doreen donated a billion of her bone marrow cells. Injected into David's abdomen, they miraculously found their way to his bone marrow, and for the first time in his life David was making antibodies. There were days in the year ahead when there was grave doubt about lasting success of the transplant, but every crisis was overcome, and the final result in this medical first was a triumph.

His sister's cells continue to produce generation after generation of new lymphocytes (the white blood cells involved in fighting infections). Indeed, they are so well established that the chromosomes in his lymphocytes are XX—female. His red blood cells, also produced in his bone marrow, are no longer his original group A but his sister's group O.

Genetically David is like the mythical fantasy—a chimera. He has one set of cells with which he was born and another functioning set donated by his sister. Phenotypically, however, he is all boy, holding his own with his friends on the playground as well as against his foes of infection in his body. David is one of fifty genetic chimeras. At least sixteen, like David, now have a system of immunity denied by nature but replaced by a feat of cellular engineering.

Another victory in the treatment of genetic disorders came closer to reality in the summer of 1973, when National Institutes of Health researcher Dr. Roscoe O. Brady reported the first success in direct replacement of a deficient enzyme. The condition is Fabry's disease, a rare sex-linked disorder affecting only males who inherit the defective gene on the X chromosome transmitted by the mother. The problem is an inability to break down fats properly owing to the enzyme deficiency. By the time the victim is in his forties fatty accumulation in the kidneys may be fatal.

When Dr. Brady injected the purified enzyme (painstakingly extracted from human placenta) into two patients, he succeeded in lowering the fat levels in their blood. For the enzyme to be effective, however, it must be administered on a sustained basis in much the same way that a diabetic gets insulin. Sufficient quantities of the enzymes are still very hard to come by, but Dr. Brady and his associates view the future with optimism not only for victims of Fabry's, but for tens of thousands of others whose genetic defects are associated with missing or deficient enzymes.

Research scientists are not alone in grappling with problems posed by the new genetics. Will successful treatment of hitherto crippling and fatal disorders increase the incidence of defective genes in the population? How should the genetic counselor deal with information he gathers from an affected family? Does he limit himself solely to imparting the information, or does he, as Dr. Pearson suggests with Huntington's disease (Chapter 16), take a more aggressive stance? What is the counselor's responsibility to other members of the family who should also know? How far, if at all, should society intervene when the risks are known and the burden of the defective child eventually is shifted to the community? (A speaker at a 1970 Down's syndrome symposium estimated that at the present rate at least $36 billion will have been spent by 1989 on institutional care for that disorder alone.)

Another new word has entered the vocabulary—bioethics. On the East Coast the Institute of Society, Ethics and the Life Sciences, Hastings, New York, and on the West Coast the Council for Biology in Human Affairs of the Salk Institute, La Jolla, California, as well as theologians, lawyers, philosophers, and scientists all over the country, are addressing themselves to questions raised by genetics, death and dying, population control, and medical ethics.

Dilemmas are also faced by parents who seek and receive genetic counseling. While amniocentesis continues to bring new hope and reassurance to thousands of families at risk, it raises soul-searching problems for others. Should a mother who knows that she is a carrier for hemophilia or Duchenne's disease (a sex-linked muscular dystrophy) choose abortion for a male fetus knowing there is a fifty-fifty chance that she may be carrying a normal baby? For the minority whose religious beliefs preclude abortion the conflicts may be even greater.

The right to abortion, a crucial tool in successful genetic counseling, is under serious threat in the United States today. No sooner did the U.S. Supreme Court hand down its historic ruling on abortion in January, 1973, than forces dedicated to wiping out the newly won rights for millions of American women went into action. The Justices said that a decision for an abortion in the first thirteen weeks of pregnancy is a matter between a woman and her physician, allowing individual states to regulate abortion later in pregnancy only when the mother's health is involved.

Some states soon passed abortion laws much more restrictive than those on the books before the Court decision. Two bills introduced into Congress later in the year threaten to reinstitute almost total prohibition. While support among legislators is still not widespread, "right to life" groups are extremely active. Should they succeed, not only will all women be deprived of access to safe legitimate abortion, but mothers seeking escape from genetic disaster may find help more difficult, if not impossible, to obtain.

Society has a special responsibility in preserving the genetic integrity of the healthy. It has been known for many years that radiation can cause mutations. When the damage is to somatic cells, the individual is affected only in his lifetime. Mutations in the germ cells (egg and sperm), on the other hand, can be carried over to succeeding generations. Although man has evolved in the presence of radioactivity—cosmic rays from outer space and radioactive natural sources on earth—modern technology has unleashed amounts of far greater magnitude. Medical and dental devices, nuclear weapons, and nuclear industrial applications are adding to the danger daily.

A significant number of new chemicals in our environment also have mutagenic powers. Drugs, notably LSD, have been associated with chromosome changes, although the evidence to date is not yet clear-cut since many LSD users are also exposed to a variety of factors known to cause chromosome breaks, including viral infections, X rays, and other drugs, each with its own unknown impurities.

A quarter of a million babies are born each year in the United States with a significant birth defect. About 20 percent of these are thought to be hereditary and another 20 percent due solely to the environment before birth, such as drugs, hormones, German measles, and other viral infections. The other 60 percent are probably due to the interactions between vulnerable genes and the environment. While the genes remain unchanged after birth, the environment throughout life does not. Vulnerable genes at birth become more vulnerable in a world with increasing hazards.

If the environment is permitted to deteriorate to the extent that damage can occur to the germ cells, that would constitute "genetic engineering" in the most negative sense. Is there "genetic engineering" in a positive sense? While there is widespread agreement that gene therapy—healing a defect in somatic cells for the lifetime of the individual—is a worthwhile goal, tampering with hereditary material (the accepted definition of genetic engineering today) will serve no useful purpose either to society or to the individual today.

The growing importance of genetics in medicine is evidenced in the increasing numbers of medical schools that give it a new prominence in their curricula. In June, 1972, the National Institutes of Health, National Institute of General Medical Sciences, awarded almost $5,000,000 in research grants to seven genetic centers that will combine both basic research and clinical studies of patients and their families. They will be looking at bone and blood disorders, heart disease, and various metabolic deficiencies.

The trend to smaller families will inevitably spare some families a child with genetic disease, even among those parents not yet aware of the danger because they have been lucky with earlier pregnancies. Meanwhile, parents at risk whose families are not yet complete are the strongest proponents of the advances in genetics and genetic counseling. Indeed, many are dedicated to spreading the message of the benefits already here and pleading for understanding and funds for the tasks still ahead.

It is a safe guess that a how-to book on genetics, written when their children are ready for parenthood, will have quite a different table of contents, showing many diseases, a problem today, to have by then been conquered.

Suggestions for Further Reading

Unraveling the Mystery of Heredity

BEADLE, GEORGE and MURIEL, *The Language of Life*. Garden City, New York, Doubleday & Company, Inc., 1966.

BOREK, ERNEST, *The Code of Life*. New York and London, Columbia University Press, 1965.

CAIRNS, JOHN; STENT, GUNTHER S.; WATSON, JAMES D., editors, *Phage and the Origins of Molecular Biology*. Cold Spring Harbor Laboratory of Quantitative Biology, 1966.

CRICK, FRANCIS, *Of Molecules and Men*. Seattle and London, University of Washington Press, 1966.

DOBZHANSKY, THEODOSIUS, *Mankind Evolving*. New York, Bantam Books, 1970.

KENDREW, JOHN C., *The Thread of Life*. Cambridge, Mass., Harvard University Press, 1966.

LURIA, S. E., *Life the Unfinished Experiment*. New York, Charles Scribner's Sons, 1973.

239

PETERS, JAMES A., *Classic Papers in Genetics*. Englewood Cliffs, N.J., Prentice-Hall, Inc., 1959.

STURTEVANT, A. H., *A History of Genetics*. New York, Harper and Row, 1965.

WATSON, JAMES D. *The Double Helix*. New York, Atheneum Publishers, 1968.

The New Look of Genetic Counseling

HARRIS, MAUREEN, editor, *Early Diagnosis of Human Genetic Defects: Scientific and Ethical Considerations*. HEW Publication No. (NIH) 72-25. Washington, D.C., Superintendent of Documents, U.S. Government Printing Office, 1972.

Sickle Cell Disease

CERAMI, ANTHONY, and WASHINGTON, ELSIE, *Sickle Cell Anemia*. New York, The Third Press, Joseph Okpaku Publishing Co., 1974.

LEWIS, ROGER, *Sickling State: Clinical Features in West Africa*. New York, Ghana University Press, Panther House Ltd., 1970.

Rh—A Matter of Incompatibility

ZIMMERMAN, DAVID R., *Rh: The Intimate History of a Disease and Its Conquest*. New York, Macmillan Publishing Co., Inc., 1973.

Pharmacogenetics

DEAN, GEOFFREY, *The Porphyrias: A Story of Inheritance and Environment*. Philadelphia, J. B. Lippincott, 1972.

240

Hemophilia

McKusick, Victor A. "The Royal Hemophilia," *Scientific American* (August, 1965).

Wilson's Disease

Greenblatt, Augusta, "What You Should Know About Inborn Diseases," *Family Circle* (April, 1967).

IQ—Are You Born to Be Smart or Stupid?

King, James C., *The Biology of Race.* New York, Harcourt Brace Jovanovich, Inc., 1971.

Senna, Carl, editor, *The Fallacy of IQ.* New York, The Third Press, Joseph Okpaku Publishing Co., Inc., 1973.

Yahraes, Herbert, *The Effect of Childhood Influences Upon Intelligence, Personality, and Mental Health.* Mental Health Program Reports-3. Public Health Service Publication No. 1876. January, 1969.

Schizophrenia—A Distorted Reality

Bleuler, Manfred, *The Offspring of Schizophrenics.* Schizophrenia Bulletin. National Institute of Mental Health. Spring, 1974.

Hawkins, David, and Pauling, Linus, editors, *Orthomolecular Psychiatry: Treatment of Schizophrenia.* San Francisco, W. H. Freeman and Company, 1972.

Mosher, Loren R.; Gunderson, John G.; Buchsbaum, Sherry, *Special Report on Schizophrenia: 1972.* Schizophrenia Bulletin. National Institute of Mental Health. Winter, 1973.

Megavitamin Therapy—Some Personal Accounts. Two letters. Schizophrenia Bulletin. National Institute of Mental Health. Winter, 1973.

Schizophrenia—Is There an Answer? DHEW Publication No. (HSM) 72-9070. 1972.

241

SNYDER, SOLOMON, *Madness and the Brain.* New York, McGraw-Hill Book Co., 1974.

The Many Faces of Mania and Melancholy

GATTOZZI, ANTOINETTE A., *Lithium in the Treatment of Mood Disorders.* National Clearinghouse for Mental Health Information Publication No. 5033. 1970.

ROSEN, GEORGE *Madness in Society.* New York, Harper and Row, Publishers, Inc., 1968.

SECUNDA, STEVEN K., et al., *The Depressive Disorders. Special Report: 1973.* National Institute of Mental Health, 1973.

The Future—Promises and Problems

BERGSMA, DANIEL; BORGAONKAR, DIGAMBER; and SHAH, SALEM, editors, *Advances in Human Genetics and Their Impact on Society.* White Plains, New York, National Foundation March of Dimes, 1972.

ETZIONI, AMITAI, *Genetic Fix.* New York, The Macmillan Co., Inc., 1974.

For Birth Defects (both hereditary and those associated with pregnancy and delivery.)

APGAR, VIRGINIA, and BECK, JOAN, *Is My Baby All Right?: A Guide to Birth Defects.* New York, Trident Press, 1972.

Where to Find Help

American Academy of Pediatrics
1801 Hinman Avenue
Evanston, Illinois 60204

American College of Obstetricians and Gynecologists
79 West Monroe Street
Chicago, Illinois 60603

Association for the Aid of Crippled Children
345 East 46th Street
New York, New York 10017

Center for Sickle Cell Anemia
College of Medicine
Howard University
520 "W" Street NW
Washington, D.C. 20001

Committee to Combat Huntington's Disease-CCHD
200 West 57th Street
New York, New York 10019

Cooley's Anemia Blood and Research Foundation for Children
3366 Hillside Avenue
New Hyde Park, New York 11040

Dysautonomia Association
608 Fifth Avenue
New York, New York 10020

Foundation for Research and Education in Sickle Cell Disease
421–431 West 120th Street
New York, New York 10027

Joseph P. Kennedy Jr. Foundation
Suite 205, 1701 "K" Street NW
Washington, D.C. 20006

Little People of America, Inc.
P.O. Box 126
Owatonna, Minnesota 55060

Muscular Dystrophy Associations of America
1790 Broadway
New York, New York 10019

National Association for Retarded Children
2709 Avenue E, East
Arlington, Texas 76011

National Clearing House for Mental Health Information
National Institute of Mental Health
5600 Fishers Lane
Rockville, Maryland 20852

National Cystic Fibrosis Foundation
3379 Peachtree Road NE
Atlanta, Georgia 30326

National Foundation-March of Dimes
P.O. Box 2000
White Plains, New York 10602.

National Genetics Foundation
250 West 57th Street
New York, New York 10019

National Hemophilia Foundation
25 West 39th Street
New York, New York 10018

National Institute of General Medical Sciences
National Institutes of Health
Bethesda, Maryland 20014

National Tay-Sachs and Allied Diseases Association, Inc.
200 Park Avenue South
New York, New York 10003

New York League for Hard of Hearing
71 West 23rd Street
New York, New York 10010

Osteogenesis Imperfecta, Inc.
1231 May Court
Burlington, North Carolina 27215

Planned Parenthood-World Population
810 Seventh Avenue
New York, New York 10019

Index